The Waltham Book of Human–Animal Interaction:

Benefits and Responsibilities of Pet Ownership

The Waltham Book of Human–Animal Interaction:

Benefits and Responsibilities of Pet Ownership

Edited by

I. ROBINSON

*Waltham Centre For Pet Nutrition,
Melton Mowbray, Leicestershire*

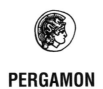

PERGAMON

U.K.	Elsevier Science Ltd., The Boulevard, Langford Lane, Kidlington, Oxford, OX5 1GB, U.K.
U.S.A.	Elsevier Science Inc., 660 White Plains Road, Tarrytown, New York 10591-5153, U.S.A.
JAPAN	Elsevier Science Japan, Tsunashima Building Annex, 3-20-12 Yushima, Bunkyo-ku, Tokyo 113, Japan

First edition 1995

Library of Congress Cataloging in Publication Data
The Waltham book of human–animal interaction: benefits and responsibilities of pet ownership/edited by I. Robinson. – 1st ed.
     p. cm.
    Includes index.
    1. Pet owners–Psychology. 2. Pets–Psychological aspects.
3. Pets–Social aspects. 4. Pets–Behavior. 5. Human–animal
relationships.   I. Robinson, I.   II. Waltham Centre for Pet
Nutrition.
SF411.47.W34   1995
636.088'7'019–dc20   95-21317

British Library Cataloguing in Publication Data
A catalogue record for this book is available from the British Library

ISBN 0 08 042284 5 (Hardcover)
ISBN 0 08 042285 3 (Flexicover)

DISCLAIMER

Whilst every effort is made by the Publishers to see that no inaccurate or misleading data, opinion or statement appear in this book, they wish to make it clear that the data and opinions appearing in the articles herein are the sole responsibility of the contributor concerned. Accordingly, the Publishers and their employees, officers and agents accept no responsibility or liability whatsoever for the consequences of any such inaccurate or misleading data, opinion or statement.

Drug and Dosage Selection: *the Authors have made every effort to ensure the accuracy of the information herein, particularly with regard to drug selection and dose. However, appropriate information sources should be consulted, especially for new or unfamiliar drugs or procedures. It is the responsibility of every veterinarian to evaluate the appropriateness of a particular opinion in the context of actual clinical situations, and with due consideration to new developments.*

Printed in Great Britain by BPC Wheatons Ltd, Exeter

Contents

Preface

The close relationship between man and animals is not a new phenomenon, but the scientific study emerged only relatively recently. However, in the last 30 years there has been a tremendous expansion in our knowledge of the behaviour of companion animals, and how humans and animals affect each other's behaviour. This information, combined with an increasingly holistic approach to health and quality of life, has led to an increase in research on how associations with animals may influence human health.

The study of human–animal interactions is a multi-disciplinary area drawing researchers from a variety of research fields. This diversity of backgrounds has caused some initial challenges as different methodological approaches and terminology are often used. Working with the authors of this book, we have attempted to clarify some of the terminology problems by using relatively strict definitions for concepts such as *"attachment"* and *"bereavement"*. Issues of differing methodological approaches can be solved by increasing communication between scientists from different backgrounds and adopting "best practice" from relevant fields.

This book is an attempt to draw together key examples of work in the area of human–animal interactions from the last 30 years, with contributions from world-wide experts in their field. The first half of this book discusses research into benefits that have been found to accrue from associations with animals, and the role of animals in care and therapy programmes. The second half considers our responsibilities toward the animals we keep, and how we can enhance their care and welfare. This section also addresses human response to pet loss. In recent years there has been an increase in interest in this area and in many countries support services exist to help pet owners during this period. However, we still lack detailed knowledge on the underlying mechanisms behind the responses, and how comparable they are to our responses to other forms of loss.

Although considerable progress in our understanding of human–animal interactions has been made, the field remains in its infancy. For the future we need to understand the mechanism behind observed effects and how these relate to our current understanding of well-being.

Acknowledgements

During the production of this book I have had help from a variety of sources. Firstly I must thank the authors for producing the chapters and their discussions regarding aspects of the text. Secondly, thanks must go to Anne McBride, Sue Ewing, and Deborah Goodwin who provided useful comments on drafts of my chapters. The support of Caroline Franklin, Fenella Bramwell, and Karen Bessant at the Grayling Company during manuscript review, and the assistance of Brenda Butler in proofreading final manuscript copy is also greatly appreciated.

List of Contributors

BEN BAARDA PhD:

Ben studied Clinical Psychology at the University of Leiden and Amsterdam, and in 1988 he received his PhD at the University of Utrecht. He is currently Associate Professor in the Department of Child Studies at the University of Utrecht, where he specialises in research methodology, especially research involving children.
Address: Department of Child Studies, University of Utrecht, Heidelberglaan 1, Utrecht, The Netherlands.

JOHN BRADSHAW BA PhD:

John graduated in Biochemistry from the University of Oxford, and obtained his PhD in animal behaviour from the University of Southampton. After 5 years as a lecturer in Biology and Chemistry at the University of Southampton, John joined the Waltham Centre for Pet Nutrition in 1983. He returned to Southampton University as a Senior Research fellow in 1987, and became Waltham Director of the Anthrozoology Institute upon its foundation in 1992. He is Honorary Secretary of the International Society for Anthrozoology, a Council member of the Association for the Study of Animal Behaviour, an Editorial Advisor to the journal *Anthrozoös* and an Honorary Scientific Advisor to the Association of Pet Behaviour Counsellors.
Address: Department of Biology, University of Southampton, Southampton, SO16 7PX, U.K.

MARY R. BURCH PhD:

Mary is the Chairperson for the Delta Society's Therapy Dog Committee and has used dogs in animal-assisted therapy settings since 1985. Her first therapy dog was the Delta Society's Therapy Animal of the Year in 1992 and her work with animal-assisted therapy and substance-exposed children has been featured in *U.S. News & World Report*, *Newsweek*, and *Reader's Digest*. In addition, Dr Burch has published numerous professional publications and has been an invited speaker on animal-assisted therapy at conferences throughout the U.S., Canada, and Mexico.
Address: Behavior Management Consultants, Inc., 2213 Napoleon Bonaparte Drive, Tallahassee, FL 32308, U.S.A.

LEO K. BUSTAD PhD DVM:

Leo is Professor and former Dean of the College of Veterinary Medicine at Washington State University (WSU). He has authored or co-authored over 200 articles, and his latest book is entitled *"Compassion: Our Last Great Hope"*. He is a member of the National Academies of Practice, a senior member of the Institute of Medicine of the National Academy of Sciences and is President Emeritus and co-founder of the Delta Society. Dr Bustad is also the 20th recipient of WSU's highest honour, The Regents Distinguished Alumnus Award.
Address: College of Veterinary Medicine, Washington State University, Pullman, WA, U.S.A.

GLYN M. COLLIS BSc PhD:

Glyn graduated from the University of Leicester in 1969 with a combined sciences degree in Psychology and Zoology, and stayed on at Leicester to do a PhD in animal behaviour. In 1972 he moved to the Department of Psychology at the University of Strathclyde to join a research group studying parent–child interaction, and in 1985 he moved to the University of Warwick as a lecturer in developmental psychology. In recent years, he has devoted much time to launching and developing a research group in Relationships, Support & Health which brings together expertise on relationships from Developmental Psychology, Social Psychology, Health Psychology & Ethology.
Address: Department of Psychology, University of Warwick, Coventry, CV4 7AL, U.K.

SUSAN DUNCAN RN:

Susan is a registered nurse who is currently a consultant for health care education and curriculum development. She is the Chairperson of the Delta Society's Service Dog Committee. She has had a variety of clinical and administrative nursing experiences related to multiple sclerosis, disability and barrier awareness, and pain aetiology. Susan has been a consultant for the research, development, and delivery of information and training regarding service dogs for people with disabilities, and has trained her own service dog which was awarded the Delta Society Service Dog of the Year Award in 1993. Ms Duncan is a lecturer on service dog issues including training, assessment and applications, legal rights, and service dogs in the workplace.
Address: c/o Delta Society, Renton, WA, U.S.A.

NIENKE ENDENBURG PhD:

Nienke completed her training in Child Psychology at the University of Utrecht in 1987, and received her PhD in 1991 for work on Human–Companion Animal Relationships at the Department of Clinical Science of Companion Animals at Utrecht University. Since then she has been studying the influence of companion animals on the development of children as a Waltham Post Doctoral Fellow at Utrecht University. In 1992 she founded the Multi-Disciplinary Research Institute on the Relationship between Humans and Animals.
Address: Department of Clinical Sciences of Companion Animals, University of Utrecht, Yalelaan 8, Utrecht, The Netherlands.

ERIKA FRIEDMANN PhD:

Erika received a doctorate in Biology from the University of Pennsylvania in 1978 and is currently Professor and Chairperson of the Department of Health and Nutrition Sciences at Brooklyn College of the City University of New York. Her classic research associating pet ownership with survival of coronary heart disease patients provided the first scientific evidence for the direct health benefits of pets and since that time she has continued researching the role of pets as mediators of stress, as well as other aspects of the roles of social and psychological factors in blood pressure, hypertension, and heart disease. Erika has published numerous scientific articles and lectured widely on this subject. She has been a member of the Delta Society since its inauguration, served on its National Research Committee, and has been president of the International Society for Anthrozoology for the past 4 years.
Address: Department of Health and Nutrition Sciences. Brooklyn College of the City University of New York, Brooklyn, NY 11210, U.S.A.

MAUREEN FREDRICKSON MSW:

Maureen is the Program Director of the Delta Society, and has been instrumental in the development and management of the Delta Pet Partners Program. She has written a workbook on clinical applications of animal-assisted therapy for human service providers and was the project co-ordinator for the Delta Society's Standards Committee that developed and published the Standards of Practice entitled "*Handbook for Animal-Assisted Activities and Animal-Assisted Therapy*". Maureen has been an invited trainer and presenter at conferences and workshops throughout the United States.
Address: c/o Delta Society, Renton, WA, U.S.A.

LYNETTE A. HART BS MA PhD:

As an undergraduate, Lynette studied Science Education at Brigham Young University and while completing an MA degree in Educational Psychology at the University of California at Berkeley, she became interested in animal behaviour. Her PhD research at Rutgers University focused on ultrasonic vocalisations associated with mating in adult rats. She then joined the Monell Chemical Senses Centre for 5 years, and subsequently worked for 1 year as a senior research scientist at American Cyanamid. Since 1982 she has been associated with the University of California, Davis, serving as the founding Director of the Center for Animals in Society at the School of Veterinary Medicine since 1985, and Director of the UC Center for Animal Alternatives since 1991. She is also an Associate Professor in the Department of Population Health and Reproduction. A primary focus of Lynette's research involves the social and lifestyle effects of interactions between humans and companion animals.
Address: Center for Animals in Society, School of Veterinary Medicine, University of California, Davis, CA 95616, U.S.A.

ANNE McBRIDE BSc PhD Cert Cons FRSA:

Anne has a degree in Psychology and a doctorate in animal behaviour from University College London. In addition to being a member of the Association of Pet Behaviour

Counsellors, holding clinics and puppy classes in the south of England, she is also Deputy Director of the Anthrozoology Institute at Southampton University. This institute specialises in the study of human–animal interactions and Anne has particular interests in several projects, including the development of separation problems in rescue dogs, temperament assessment of dogs, the role of dogs in the education of severely learning-disabled children, and the relationship between pet ownership and the general health of elderly people. She is course co-ordinator for the Postgraduate Diploma in Companion Animal Behaviour Counselling at the University of Southampton, and Deputy Chairman of "Pathway," a committee set up to review pets and housing issues in the U.K.

Address: Department of Adult Continuing Education, University of Southampton, Southampton, SO17 1BJ, U.K.

SANDRA McCUNE VN BA (Mod.) PhD:

Sandra qualified as a veterinary nurse in Dublin in 1993, later becoming a Council member of the British Veterinary Nursing Association (1991–1993). She went on to study Zoology at Trinity College, Dublin from 1984–1988 specialising in Physiology. Her final year research project looked at the transmission of ear mites between cats. In 1988 she went to Cambridge University where she completed a PhD on temperament in cats and how it influences their ability to cope with confinement. Sandra joined the Waltham Centre for Pet Nutrition in 1993 and currently works on the development of dog and cat behaviour and the relationship between cats and their owners.

Address: Waltham Centre for Pet Nutrition, Waltham-on-the-Wolds, Melton Mowbray, Leicestershire, LE14 4RT, U.K.

JUNE McNICHOLAS BSc:

June graduated from the University of Warwick in 1991 with a degree in Psychology, and as a result of her undergraduate projects in companion animal studies, she was appointed as a Research Fellow on a project investigating the issue of pet ownership for people in residential care, funded by the Joseph Rowntree Foundation. Her particular research interest is in health psychology and she is a member of the Relationships, Support and Health research group at Warwick. June is currently a Waltham Research Fellow investigating the role of pets as providers of social support, a possible explanation for the beneficial effects of pet ownership.

Address: Department of Psychology, University of Warwick, Coventry, CV4 7AL, U.K.

JUSTINE A. McPHERSON BSc:

Justine graduated in Genetics from Nottingham University in 1992, and is currently studying for a PhD at the Anthrozoology Institute, University of Southampton. Her research, on the development of attachment behaviour in dogs, is supported by the Biotechnology and Biological Sciences Research Council and the Blue Cross animal welfare charity.

Address: Department of Biology, University of Southampton, Southampton, SO16 7PX, U.K.

IAN ROBINSON BSc PhD:

Ian graduated from the University of Durham in 1983 with a degree in Zoology and obtained his PhD, studying olfactory communication in carnivores, from the University of Aberdeen in 1987. Ian joined the Waltham Centre for Pet Nutrition in 1988 as an animal behaviourist, studying the feeding behaviour of dogs and cats, and in his current position he is involved in studies of pet–owner relationships, focusing on how both human and animal behaviour can influence the relationship. He is a committee member of the Society for Companion Animal Studies and the International Society for Anthrozoology and is particularly interested in the health benefits that are associated with pet ownership.
Address: Waltham Centre for Pet Nutrition, Waltham-on-the-Wolds, Melton Mowbray, Leicestershire, LE14 4RT, U.K.

JEAN TEBAY MS:

Jean has been a Board Member of the Federation of Riding for the Disabled International, and was the Chairperson of the Delta Society's Committee to develop standards for animal-assisted therapy. She has worked extensively in the area of therapeutic riding in conjunction with Therapeutic Riding Services, and has been a long time supporter of the need for standards, a curriculum, and research focusing on therapeutic riding. She has been an invited presenter at therapeutic riding conferences throughout the United States.
Address: c/o Delta Society, Renton, WA, U.S.A.

DENNIS C. TURNER Dr sc:

Dennis is director of the Institute for Applied Ethology and Animal Psychology in Hirzel and president of the Konrad Lorenz Trust, IEMT-Switzerland. He is a Vice-President of the International Association of Human Animal Interaction Organisations (I.A.H.A.I.O.), Program Chairman of the 7th international conference on human–animal interactions, "*Animals, Health & Quality of Life*," in Geneva, 1995, European editor of *Anthrozoös*, and the Companion Animal Section editor for *Animal Welfare*. Together with Patrick Bateson, he edited *The Domestic Cat: The Biology of its Behaviour*. Dennis is a "certified applied animal behaviourist" (U.S. Animal Behavior Society), a member of the Association of Pet Behaviour Counsellors in London and of the professional pet behaviour counsellor societies V.H.V.T.S. and V.I.E.T.A. in Switzerland. He is also chief advisor on companion animal behaviour problems at the Small Animal Clinic, Veterinary School, University of Zürich.
Address: I.E.T. Postfach 32, CH-8816 Hirzel, Switzerland.

CHAPTER 1

Associations Between Man and Animals

IAN ROBINSON

Introduction

In the last few years there has been a tremendous increase in interest in relationships between man and animals and in particular with the animals we keep as companions. This has generated a substantial amount of research and a number of extensive reviews of historical attitudes to, and associations with, animals.[10,15,17,18] This chapter does not aim to duplicate these reviews but will provide a brief overview of man's association with animals and our relationship with companion animals. Later chapters will then discuss two of the most important aspects of this relationship, namely the benefits we receive from companion animals and our responsibilities to them.

Animals in Human Societies

Animals have been a key aspect of human life for many thousands of years. From earliest human times they have been important for the provision of food and as a focus for religious worship. When thinking about primal human communities and their interactions

with animals, we tend to consider animals mainly as a source of food, or perhaps a means of transport or providers of agricultural power. In developing nations, this traditional use is still in evidence. However, in the developed world the role of many animals in society has changed. Although animals are still used as a source of food, even this practice is declining with the increase in vegetarianism. Perhaps surprisingly it has been discovered that pet-keeping is not merely a phenomenon of the relatively affluent western world, but is widespread in other cultures[12,15–18] and is an ancient activity, older than the domestication of animals for food and transport needs.

Early Hunting Communities

The young of many mammal species were tamed and kept in captivity by Palaeolithic people, at least for short periods of time. Whether these animals remained tame as adults would depend on the social behaviour of the species.[1] Clutton-Brock[1] suggests that the taming of young wolves is likely to have occurred in many parts of the world as early

1

as 500 thousand years ago. Other carnivores would also have been tamed, but associations with wolves could continue as the animals matured because of similarities between human and wolf social systems. Wolves and humans were competitors for ungulate prey and it is possible that man used tame wolves for their ability to detect and track prey. There are other possibilities for the initial role of tame wolves in human society. Studies of Australian aborigines have shown that tame dingoes are only effective as cooperative hunters in tropical rain forests and the main value of the dingo is to keep the camp clean of rubbish, to keep humans warm at night and to give warning of intruders.[9] Thus, wolves may not have been efficient hunting aids for early man.

Whatever the initial reason for taking wolves from the wild, selection of those wolves best suited to living with man would eventually have led to the domestication of the wolf, leading to the development of the modern dog. Apart from the utilitarian role proposed for dogs, there is early evidence to suggest that they were also considered as companions. In Northern Israel, a 12,000-year-old Palaeolithic tomb was uncovered which contained the remains of a human and a dog buried together. The dead person's hand had been arranged so that it rested on the animal's shoulder, as if to emphasise a bond that had existed between the two individuals during life.[2]

Historical reviews of humans and their attitudes to animals show how our perceptions have changed over the centuries.[10] Before man refined agricultural techniques and became settled, the traditional lifestyle was one of hunting and gathering. An insight into the relationships of hunter–gatherer communities with animals can be gained from reviews of historical texts or studying contemporary hunter–gatherer communities.[8] Between the 16th and 19th centuries, European missionaries and explorers of the New World reported a variety of animal species kept as companions.[17] They described how native peoples often refused to part with their animals, even for payment, and were

distressed if the animals were forcibly removed. Accounts of this pet-keeping practice usually express ridicule or astonishment at the degree of affection demonstrated for these animals, indicating that close relationships with animals were not common in Europe at that time.

Pet-keeping in hunter–gatherer societies produced no conflicts with the hunting lifestyle, as all animals were treated with respect.[8] Animals were considered to have souls which the hunter could release and were thought to offer themselves to be killed only if the hunter treated them or their fellow animals with respect. It is possible that caring for a few members of a species may have been seen as a way of earning respect from their wild counterparts and thus improve hunting success,[3] although this would not explain the presence of animals of species not hunted for food. However, it is possible that primitive man was able to consider animals purely as companions far earlier than current evidence suggests.

The Development of Farming Communities

The gradual change to settled agriculture, which took place in some human communities around 10,000 years ago, led to a change in human perception of animals. Farming practices involved keeping wild animals away from crops, whilst animals intended for human consumption were restrained to prevent them from roaming. Thus, human attitudes to many animal species shifted from the respect and trust shown by hunter–gatherers, to one of domination.[8] Close associations between man and newly domesticated animals also led to the incorporation of animals into religious and cultural activities. In many ancient civilizations certain animal species were seen to share important characteristics with humans, but in exaggerated forms which inspired admiration or fear. The most culturally significant of these were those species perceived as representing power or domination and libido or fertility. Cattle were domesticated early by agricultural man and therefore bovine images became particularly important.[14]

Domestication of the cat began with the development of settled agriculture in Egypt. Initially, small wild felids are likely to have scavenged around human communities, feeding upon vermin attracted to food stores. From about 5000 years ago the Egyptians confined cats in temples for religious purposes and no doubt there was selection for the most friendly individuals. Around 3000 years ago there was a gradual secularisation of cat-keeping in Egypt and an associated trade in cats to other countries, despite attempts by the Egyptian authorities to prevent this.[19]

Representations of dogs also featured in some ancient civilisations, usually associated with death. In some cases the deceased were deliberately put out for dogs to consume, as it was thought that the soul of the deceased must pass through a dog to reach the afterlife. These early associations between dogs and death gradually evolved into beliefs that dogs could ward off or prevent death. The Greeks thought that dogs had the ability to cure illness and kept them as co-therapists in their healing temples.[14]

The horse entered many ancient cultures too late to assume the religious significance of cattle, but once introduced it became very important. The horse provided the rulers of cattle-rich states with a source of speed and stamina in excess of that available from cattle. As Greek and Roman civilisations developed, the ancient beliefs about the power of cattle began to fade and they became utilitarian possessions. The prestige associated with cattle was transferred to the horse.

As civilisations developed, human–animal relationships became more peripheral and symbolic, and with this came the increasing view that man had dominion over all animals. These ideas were developed further by religious and secular teachings. For example, Greek philosophy considered mankind to be at the top of a natural hierarchy and the biblical view was that man had God-given dominion over the rest of creation. Although animals lost much of their religious and cultural

importance, some animals remained closely associated with man, albeit subtly, in the role of companions.

Animals as Companions

Historical Associations

The keeping of animals purely as companions may appear to be a modern phenomenon, but pet ownership by the ruling or noble classes has a long history. Ancient Egyptian murals show pharaohs keeping companion animals. Many generations of Chinese emperors kept dogs, which as puppies were often suckled by human wet nurses and as adults were tended to by their own servants.[15] Greek and Roman nobility were also avid keepers of pets.

In mediaeval Europe, pet-keeping was recorded amongst the European aristocracy and by members of the church.[12,18] The Christian church frowned upon this practice, suggesting that the food used for these animals should be given to the poor. However, fears that close associations with animals were strongly linked to pagan worship are a more likely explanation for this condemnation. The prejudice against pets reached its height during the Inquisition where evidence against heretics often included references to close associations with animals. Reports of associations with animals as companions occurred during witch trials, where the possession of an 'animal familiar' was used as evidence of witchcraft.[18] Many of the people accused of witchcraft were elderly and socially isolated women, suggesting that they kept animals for the benefit of companionship.

The most likely reason for negative attitudes to companion animals for much of history was because affectionate relationships towards animals were considered to be immoral and against the natural order of life. Pet-keeping by the privileged elite was facilitated by their wealth and rank which meant that they could afford to keep non-working animals and ignore criticism of the practice. However, even amongst the elite there was little regard for the welfare of animals in general. This is because until relatively recently there was a commonly held view in the western world that animals lacked feelings and were created in order to serve humanity.[7]

Pet-keeping amongst a wider European population did not begin to acquire acceptance until the end of the 17th century and widespread pet-keeping amongst the middle classes did not become a common phenomenon until the late 18th century. It has been argued that pet-keeping in its present form is a 19th-century Victorian invention,[12] prompted by a change in mankind's perception of his position in the world. As the natural world became increasingly explored, understood and mastered, pet-keeping became a link with a natural world which itself was no longer seen as threatening. It also allowed a visible demonstration of man's domination over nature. For example, in the development of new breeds, the breeder assumed an almost god-like role in the search for new variations and the control of animal reproduction. However, the practice of pet-keeping also reflected other social attitudes of the time. Pet-keeping by the 'lower classes' was seen as inappropriate as it was considered to encourage the neglect of other social duties. Pets were therefore defined as an inappropriate luxury for the 'lower classes', who lacked the moral means to control them and the financial means to support them.[12]

Modern Pet-keeping

Present day attitudes to animals vary considerably across the world. For example, in India the cow is a sacred animal allowed to wander at will and its slaughter and consumption are forbidden. In western societies, however, cows are utilised for milk, meat and leather; cats and dogs are given many of the privileges of Indian cows. In contrast, in some parts of the Far East dogs and cats are used for food. Most research on interactions between companion animals and man has been conducted in western societies. These studies therefore tend to concentrate on western attitudes to animals and on the customary western pets.

Pets can have a number of functions ranging from ornamental to status symbol, from helpers to companions. Exotic birds and fish may have a purely ornamental role and in many parts of Southern Europe songbirds may be kept for their ornamental value in cages hanging outside houses. Pets can also act as a channel for personal expression. People express their personality in a variety of ways, the clothes they choose, the car they drive and the type of pet they own. For example, the person who chooses a breed of dog perceived by society as aggressive may be using that dog as a way of acting out their own hostile feelings towards society.[11,13,20] Likewise, owners of exotic or dangerous pets (such as poisonous snakes and spiders) may be making a statement about their status, along the lines that only someone powerful and independent could own such an animal.

Pet-keeping as a hobby is also relatively common in the western world and the practice varies from the very popular activity of showing and breeding animals such as pedigree cats and dogs, to the keeping of certain strains of fish or birds as a collection. Where animals are kept as a form of collection, relationships may not be formed with individual animals but rather with some distinct aspect of the species or breed which is divorced from the individual animal's character. In this way the animals can be used to make some statement about the owner or be an instrument by which the owner can interact with other people.

Human–Animal Relationships

The most common reason for pet ownership in western societies is companionship. This activity differs from most other forms of ownership in that its primary aim is the complex relationship that can develop. Whereas most domesticated animals provide economic or practical benefits, the rewards from keeping animals as companions are derived from the relationship itself. However, this does not exclude the possibility that people who keep animals for other reasons also develop strong relationships with their animals.

The reasons people develop relationships with animals are various and reflect the human's personality and attitudes.[20] The relationship that develops with companion animals is comparable to that which develops between human companions and can vary in intensity and form in a similar way. The differences in types of relationship may be due to variations in the behavioural characteristics of either the humans or the animals involved. Appropriate socialisation, positive experiences and prolonged physical contact can all facilitate the establishment of a bond between animal and human.[4,5] In addition, the more similar the social organisation and communication systems of the two species, the more likely that each will recognise signals from the other and be able to respond appropriately.[6] This similarity, especially with regard to communication and sensory systems, tends to be greater between the 'higher' vertebrates and humans and therefore we are more likely to have a closer relationship with a dog or a cat than we are with a fish or a reptile. Dogs and cats are unique among domestic animals in that they retain association with man without being caged or tethered. This may partially explain their popularity as pets. As demonstrated by the chapters in this book, they have also been the focus for most of the research into human–animal interactions.

A popular perception of pet ownership among many non-owners is that pets are child substitutes or inferior replacements for human social interactions. Pet owners may therefore be thought of as socially or emotionally inadequate. Whilst this view may be true in a few cases, many studies have shown that the majority of pet owners are normal people whose companion animals improve existing human social relationships (see *Chapters 2 and 3*). Until recently it was thought that benefits from companion animal or pet ownership were confined to the fulfilment of emotional or social needs. However, as detailed in chapters of this book, benefits

of pet ownership have now been shown to include improvements in psychological and physiological health. This, combined with the fact that pet-keeping is a common phenomenon in many societies, including those with a fragile economic base, suggests that our association with other species fulfils a need which goes beyond simple economic considerations.

References

1. Clutton-Brock, J. (1994) The unnatural world: behavioural aspects of humans and animals in the process of domestication. In *Animals and Human Society: Changing Perspectives*. Eds. A. Manning and J. Serpell. pp. 23–35. Routledge, London.
2. Davis, J. M. and Valla, F. R. (1978) Evidence for domestication of the dog 12,000 years ago in the Natufian of Israel. *Nature*, **276,** 608–610.
3. Erikson, P. (1987) De l'apprivoisement a l'approvisionnement. Chasse, alliance et familiarisation en Amazonie Amerindienne. *Techniques et Cultures*, **9,** 105–140.
4. Estep, D. Q. and Hetts, S. (1992) Interactions, relationships and bonds: the conceptual basis for scientist–animal relations. In *The Inevitable Bond*. Eds. H. Davis and D. Balfour. pp. 6–26. Cambridge University Press.
5. Fentress, J. (1992) The covalent animal: on bonds and their boundaries in behavioural research. In *The Inevitable Bond*. Eds. H. Davis and D. Balfour. pp. 44–71. Cambridge University Press.
6. Hediger, H. (1965) Man as a social partner of animals and vice-versa. In *Symposia of the Zoological Society of London*. Ed. P. E. Ellis. Vol. 14, pp. 291–300
7. Hume, C. W. (1957) *The Status of Animals in the Christian Religion*. Universities Federation for Animal Welfare, Potters Bar, Middlesex.
8. Ingold, T. (1994) From trust to domination: an alternative history of human–animal relations. In *Animals and Human Society: Changing Perspectives*. Eds. A. Manning and J. Serpell. pp. 1–22. Routledge, London.
9. Meggitt, M. J. (1965) The association between Australian aborigines and dingoes. In *Man, Culture and Animals*. Eds. A. Leeds and A. P. Vayada. pp. 7–26. AAAS Publication 78, Washington, DC.
10. Manning, A. and Serpell, J. (Eds.) (1994) *Animals and Human Society: Changing Perspectives*. Routledge, London.
11. O'Farrell, V. (1994) *Dogs' Best Friend*. Methuen.

12. Ritvo, H. (1988) The emergence of modern pet-keeping. In *Animals and People Sharing the World.* Ed. A. N. Rowan. pp. 13–32. University Press of New England, Hanover, USA.

13. Rosenbaum, J. (1972) *Is Your Volkswagen a Sex Symbol?* Bantam, New York.

14. Schwabe, C. W. (1994) Animals in the ancient world. In *Animals and Human Society: Changing Perspectives.* Eds. A. Manning and J. Serpell. pp. 36–58. Routledge, London

15. Serpell, J. A. (1986) *In the Company of Animals: A Study of Human–Animal Relationships.* Basil Blackwell Ltd, Oxford.

16. Serpell, J. (1987) Pet-keeping in non-western societies: some popular misconceptions. *Anthrozoös,* **1**(3), 166–174.

17. Serpell, J. (1988) Pet-keeping in non-western societies: some popular misconceptions. In *Animals and People Sharing the World.* Ed. A. N. Rowan. pp. 33–52. University Press of New England, Hanover, USA.

18. Serpell, J. and Paul, E. (1994) Pets and the development of positive attitudes to animals. In *Animals and Human Society: Changing Perspectives.* Eds. A. Manning and J. Serpell. pp. 127–144. Routledge, London

19. Thorne, C. (1992) Evolution and domestication. In *The Waltham Book of Dog and Cat Behaviour.* Ed. C. Thorne. pp. 1–30. Pergamon Press, Oxford.

20. Veevers, J. E. (1985) The social meaning of pets: Alternative roles for companion animals. In *Pets and the Family.* Ed. M. Sussman. *Marriage and Family Review,* **8,** 11–30.

CHAPTER 2

The Role of Pets in Enhancing Human Well-being: Effects on Child Development

NIENKE ENDENBURG and BEN BAARDA

Introduction

Parents often obtain a pet because they consider them to be good for their children. These parents will state that their children become more responsible, are more sociable and develop character.[26] However, the relationship between humans and animals and especially the influence of pets on children is a relatively new area for scientific research. One of the first to investigate this area was the American child psychologist Boris Levinson.[33] Levinson worked with a boy who had many problems associated with social contact. On one occasion Levinson happened to have his dog with him in the office. The dog was not usually permitted into the office when clients were expected, but on this day the boy arrived earlier than expected for his appointment. The boy began to interact with the dog and to Levinson's surprise spoke to the dog; Levinson had not been able to provoke speech during the previous month. This was the beginning of his research, which has inspired many others to investigate this area.

Early studies were mainly case studies, later followed by questionnaire, survey and interview approaches. Although a considerable number of interesting studies have since been reported, the mechanisms that lie behind the results obtained remain unclear.

One of the problems is that it is difficult to conduct experimental research in this area. For example it is not possible to force people to take a pet while others are told that they cannot own one. It is therefore difficult to say anything about causal relationships. Sometimes in childrens' homes it is possible to give an animal to certain groups, while other similar groups do not get one, but this kind of study is rare and it is difficult to generalise these data to children living with their families under 'normal' circumstances. To overcome the problem of causality, longitudinal studies can be conducted but these are time consuming and expensive.[26]

Despite these difficulties, some research has been carried out on the question of whether or not pets have an influence on the development of children. Melson and Peet[40]

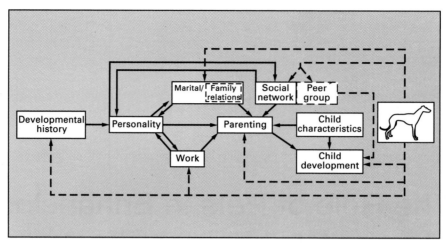

FIG. 2.1: A process model of the determinants of child development and the possible influence of pets.

found that being attached to a pet is related to positive emotional functioning. Bergesen[10] affirmed this and wrote that it is the positive self-esteem of children that is enhanced by owning a pet. According to Poresky and Hendrix,[46] it is not only social–emotional development, but also cognitive development that can be enhanced by owning pets. In these and other studies it was possible to measure relationships and to demonstrate that there were some effects, yet the mechanisms that lie behind these effects did not attract much attention. Theoretical implications to be drawn from these investigations could provide more insight into the mechanisms which cause these effects.

During the last decade of developmental psychology there has been more attention paid to why some children fail to develop properly under severe circumstances while others develop well. Several models have evolved to take account of the variables that influence the development of children.[1,9,50–52] Although these models have much in common, they concentrate on different aspects of development and the variables that influence that development. This chapter gives an explanatory outline of child development and the variables that influence that development. The research conducted on the influence of pets on the development of children will be reviewed with reference to Belsky's model.[9]

The Development of Children

Child development is an ongoing process. Children have to master tasks concerning cognitive development, as well as social and emotional development. There are several variables influencing this development. In Belsky's model[9] three domains of variables are identified: the characteristics of the child, personal psychological resources of the parents and contextual sources of stress and support. These domains interact with each other and will determine how the child will develop. A differentiation can be made between 'child characteristics' and 'child development'. In the domain of personal psychological resources of the parents the 'personality', the 'work', the 'marital relations' and the 'parenting style' are important factors and in the domain of contextual sources of stress and support 'social network' and 'peer group' and also 'housing conditions', can be important.

A child's characteristics include genetically determined factors such as temperament and intelligence. These factors influence the development of the child, but as they are relatively stable and cannot be influenced to a great extent by other variables such as parenting, they will not be discussed further.

Child development consists of both social–emotional development and cognitive development. Social–emotional development can be measured by self-esteem and a positive social orientation of the child, but social skills and a sense of social or moral responsibility can also contribute to the building of self-esteem. The level of cognitive development can be examined, when children learn to read, write and are able to do mathematics. The development of the child is also influenced by the social network of that child. For instance if the child has no friends their social development will be different from a child who has many friends. Cochran and Brassard[20] found that the support provided by social networks can enhance self-esteem. There is considerable evidence that effective social support contributes to mental health and some evidence that it may provide a buffering, protective function against psychosocial stress.[21,44]

Parents are very important in the life of a child, therefore parenting will influence the development of that child. Parental use of induction or reasoning, consistent discipline and expression of warmth have been found to relate positively to self-esteem and intellectual achievement during the school-age years.[9] Parents should also be sensitive to the needs of their children. The model of parental functioning assumes that there is a link between parents' psychological well-being and their parental functioning that can be traced back to the parents' own experiences while growing up. The developmental history of the parents will thus influence their personality. Other factors such as marital relations also influence parenting. It has been found that marital is the most important form of support and Belsky[8] found that a positive marital relationship is a major supporting factor in competent parenting. This model can be extended by adding family relations and cohesion, in cases where family members are able to rely on each other and feel that accepted stressful experiences can be resolved together.

Apart from the beneficial effect of social support on the development of children, social networks can also have a beneficial influence on parenting. One of the reasons social networks are important is that they provide emotional support. This support can be defined as the love and interpersonal acceptance an individual receives from others, either through explicit statements to that effect or as a result of considerate actions,[9] so that people feel cared for and accepted.

The work status of the parents is the last variable included in Belsky's model, that can influence parenting. Unemployment can introduce a level of stress into the family and will also influence the financial status.[3] If both parents work, the children may have other forms of daytime care, although there is no evidence that this has a significant negative or positive influence on their development.[31]

Having briefly discussed this model, it is important to remember that there will be other variables influencing the development of the child which are not mentioned in this model. However, we consider this model to be the most useful framework for examining the potential influence of pets on the development of children. It is also important to realise that the aforementioned variables are not independent but influence each other. For instance, parenting influences the social–emotional development of the child but this in turn influences parenting. Thus, the development of children is a dynamic process whose key feature lies in the process, not in the variable. There is a danger that researchers may concentrate on the variables rather than on the mechanisms involved.[55] For pragmatic reasons, however, only the different variables in this relationship will be examined in this chapter.

Direct Influences of Pets on the Development of Children

Child development can be separated into social–emotional and cognitive development. First the direct influences will be discussed, starting with social–emotional development.

Social–Emotional Development

There is scientific evidence that self-esteem is an important aspect of the social–emotional

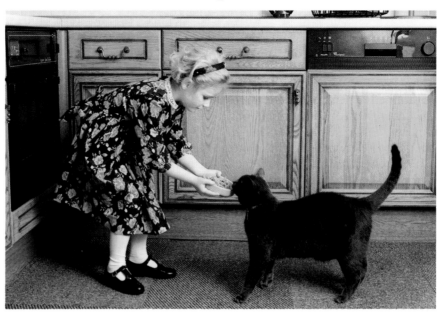

Fig. 2.2: Children should be given pet care tasks that are appropriate to
their age.

development of children.[30,50] If there are pets in the house, parents and children frequently share in taking care of the pet, which suggests that youngsters learn at an early age how to care for and nurture a dependent animal.[29] For younger children, involvement, positive reinforcement and acceptance are important for building self-esteem. Accomplishing tasks appropriate to their age, when taking care of the pet with their parents, makes a child feel more competent. However, this process relies on parents knowing which tasks are appropriate. A 3-year-old cannot walk a dog, but can help with giving a dog water. If parents are aware of this fact, children receive positive reinforcement from their parents when they take care of an animal in a responsible way. As the child grows older the allocation of responsibility for pet-care management changes in a child-centred family. Pre-school children enjoy imitating their parent's work, whereas the school-age child can manage some tasks alone and the teenager independently can assume certain responsibilities. Bergesen[10] found that children's self-esteem scores increased significantly over a nine month period of keeping pets in their school class-

room. In particular, it was children with originally low self-esteem scores who showed the greatest improvements. Covert *et al.*[24] found that early adolescent pet owners had higher self-esteem scores than non-pet owners. Davis[25] found a significant positive association between pre-adolescents' affective relationships with the family dog and their perceived self-concept.

Another aspect of social–emotional development is empathy, the child's ability to understand how someone else feels. According to Paul[45] it is possible that by interacting with pets that are totally dependent on the owner, children learn to understand the feelings and needs of animals and those of fellow human beings from an early age. Bryant[14] found that children who owned pets felt more empathy towards other people. Poresky and Hendrix[47] also found that 3–6-year-old pet-owning children achieved higher empathy scores than their non-pet-owning counterparts. Ascione[2] found that an animal-based humane education programme in elementary school was related to higher empathy scores amongst fourth graders (although not amongst first, second and fifth graders). Poresky and Hendrix[48] claim that it is not owning pets *per se*, but particularly the compassion children feel towards pets, that is related to their empathy towards humans.

Pets also have been cited as providing important 'social' support.[14,27,32] Bachman[3] found that children regularly nominated pets when asked who they would go to with a problem. Brickel[13] reports that companion animals can provide emotional support. Levinson[35] believed that this sort of emotional support could be important for the healthy psychological development of all children. The 'social' support given by pets has some advantages compared to the social support given by humans. Pets can make people feel unconditionally accepted, whereas fellow humans will judge and may criticise. Ros[54] stated that social support given by other humans can be threatening.

Enduring affection is a significant source of the potential benefit and pleasure that pets can bring to children. Children sense that pets will love and accept them unconditionally (even when the child gets angry or performs poorly at school[16]) and provide a source of non-judgemental affection.[5] This does not mean that pets can replace humans. They can give emotional support, but they cannot give instrumental support, such as advice, or help with homework.

Cognitive Development

Poresky *et al.*[49] associated improved cognitive development with the bond between children and pets. It has been suggested that pet ownership might facilitate language acquisition and enhance verbal skills in children.[22,56] This would occur as a result of the pet functioning both as a patient recipient of the young child's babble and as an attractive verbal stimulus, eliciting communication from the child in the form of praise, orders, encouragement and punishment. However, no real evidence has yet been offered to support these hypotheses.[46] More research is needed to find out whether pets could have any influence on the cognitive development.

This review of the influence of pets on the development of children shows that not all studies give the same results. This may be due to the fact that not every child likes taking care of an animal, some may even be afraid. Poresky *et al.*[49] studied the attachment between the child and the pet. They found that attachment between child and pet was a more reliable measure than the owning of a pet *per se*. Melson[39] also found that attachment to pets was positively related to the self-esteem of children in kindergarten; but there was no relationship between attachment to pets and self-esteem of second (mean age 8.14 years) and fifth (mean age 12.01 years) graders. Attachment might seem to be a mediating variable between the pet and the development of the child.

Indirect Influences of Pets on the Development of Children

Parenting

Parents play an important role in pet selection since it is the attitudes of parents which determine whether there will be a pet in the household and the type of pet owned. Studies have shown that people who owned a pet in childhood are significantly more likely to own a pet as an adult.[26,45,57] People who had experience of a pet during childhood have a more positive attitude towards pets[45] and a better understanding of the non-verbal signals of such a pet.[6] Pet ownership occurs significantly more often in families with school-aged children and adolescents than in families without children.[26,42]

Many parents admit that pets can be valuable tools with which to educate children about life events.[37,56] Two such situations where parental reactions probably influence children is when an animal is born or when it dies. Children who have pets in the family will probably experience the death of an animal. This is a painful experience and the way in which their parents and others near to them deal with the situation will have an influence on how children cope with death in general throughout their lives. It is important

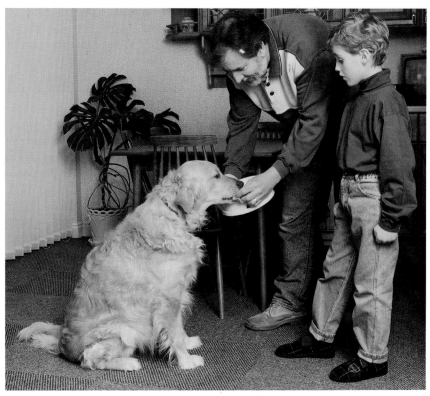

FIG. 2.3: Pet ownership occurs significantly more often in families with
children than in those without children.

for parents to discuss their feelings of sadness openly and to share the associated feelings with the child. Parents have to show that it is all right to have such feelings. Learning to cope with sad feelings, for instance when a pet dies or is euthanased, is important and parents have to help their children with it. The veterinarian can also play an important role here. To explain what happens when a pet is euthanased in a way children can understand, will help the child with the grieving process.

At the other end of an animal's life is birth. For most children the birth of animals is an exciting moment which can give parents the opportunity to explain how life begins and can form part of sex education.

Marital and Family Relations

Family influences are associated with both pet ownership/bonding and child develop-

ment. Paul[45] found significant results suggesting that dog ownership was associated with greater family cohesion. When a pet has been acquired there is an initial increase in the frequency of children's social interactions, at least within their own home. Cain[18] found that of families surveyed in the USA, 52% reported experiencing an increase in the time the family spent together after they acquired their pets. As many as 70% reported an increase in family happiness and fun subsequent to pet acquisition. These subjective data have limitations, but suggest that people believe, or at least would like to believe, that their pets enhance family cohesion and increase the time spent with each other. Thus, people believe that pets act as social facilitators within the family.

Some research has reported that pets can play a particularly important role in the lives of children who have inadequate or destructive family and social environments.[11,34,53]

However, Bryant and Whorley[17] found that children's use of their pets for emotional support was most clearly related to a good experience of such support from their parents. Poresky and Hendrix[47] also found that children with pets and a better home environment showed higher age-adjusted child development scores.[47]

Sibling status and number are also significantly related to childhood pet ownership. There is a tendency for children with fewer siblings and those with no younger siblings in particular, to have more pets of their own and to appear to be more pet-oriented.[15,38,45] Perhaps single and youngest children use animals to express feelings and perform behaviour that other children are able to direct towards their younger sisters or brothers.

Social Networks Influencing the Development of Children

Many people seem to experience social support in their interactions with animals or with other people through companion animals. Mugford and M'Comisky[43] used the term **social lubricant** to describe the phenomenon where the presence of animals increased social contacts between people. This effect has been noted by a number of others.[23,35,36,41,56] Guttman *et al.*[28] suggested that the attractiveness of a child's pet to other children may, as a secondary effect, enhance the attractiveness of the child as a friend or playmate. MacDonald[37] found that 84% of the 31 10-year-olds he interviewed reported that social contacts occurred with other children and adults while they exercised their dogs. Pet owning children have also been found to be significantly more popular with their classmates.[28] Other results suggest that adolescent pet-owners are significantly more lonely than adolescent non-owners.[7] However, it is possible that people who feel lonely obtain a pet to remedy the situation and so the issue of cause and effect remains unclear. Longitudinal studies are required to shed more light on the causal relationship and whether other variables play a mediating role.

It may not be ownership as such, but attachment to the pet which is important. Melson[39] has shown that involvement with a pet, and not simply pet ownership is related to children's involvement in non-school social activities. Further research is required to show whether or not attachment and involvement are the same concepts in this context.

Social Networks Influencing Parenting

Research has demonstrated that social support is positively related to good parental functioning. This is not surprising since social support and general well-being have been repeatedly linked. In addition to the direct social support provided by pets, they can also provide an indirect support by serving as a catalyst for social contacts with other persons for both children and parents.[23,35,36,41,56]

Parental Employment Status

Pets may play an important role when both parents are employed. It can be suggested that pets provide a constant in children's lives and that they are predictably responsive e.g. welcoming the children when they come home. Unfortunately, no research has been conducted in this area. However, the influence of pets on child development and parenting and whether this is dependent on the parents' employment status ought to be investigated.

Can Pets Enhance the Development of Children?

The aim of this chapter was to set out the way in which pets could influence the development of children. Our approach was to place published research data in a theoretical framework. It becomes clear that pets can have positive influences on certain aspects of child development. However, as stated earlier, causal relationships are difficult to prove and

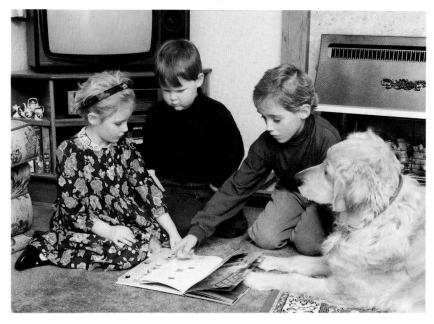

Fig. 2.4: Acquisition of a pet increases the frequency of children's social interactions within their own home.

more attention must be paid to the mechanisms behind these influences.

Research to date has not been equally distributed in the different areas of development. Areas that have been neglected include whether pets have a direct influence on the cognitive development of children, or whether parents who allow pets in their family manifest a different parental style to those who do not.

The employment status of the parents should also be taken into account when the influence of pets on the development of children is studied. It is possible that pets play different roles when both, one, or neither parent is employed.

It would be interesting to see whether children and parents who own animals have better social networks than people without animals. Both the number and the quality of contacts should be considered, since it is possible that while people with pets may have more surface contacts, the quality of social support they enjoy does not differ from people without animals.

When we talk about the development of children we also have to bear in mind both the factors that facilitate the development (protective factors) and the factors that can be a threat to this development (risk factors). From this review it appears that pets can act as protective factors, but the research reported did not consider potential negative aspects. For instance, it is possible that there may be more stress in a family where no one is willing to take care of the animal. Serpell[58] on the other hand, suggested that benefits and problems with pets and children can signal existing or impending crises within families. Therefore some consideration should be given to the potential costs of owning pets, in order to define those situations where the benefits are greater than perceived costs.

This review of the influence of pets on the development of children has made a preliminary attempt to place the research results into a theoretical framework. It can however be nothing more than a beginning. If we want to understand the mechanisms that lie behind these results we need research guided by theoretical frameworks in order to test developmental models and the roles of pets within them. The consequence of these ideas is that research must focus on all aspects of development and the pet–child relationship. Such data is important for parents, teachers and professionals working in mental and physical health care.

References

1. Abidin, R. R. (1991) Measures of parental characteristics as predictors of child behavioral adjustment and self-esteem for children 2–7 years of age. Unpublished lecture. University of Virginia, Charlottes Ville, VA.
2. Ascione, F. R. (1992) Enhancing children's attitudes about the humane treatment of animals: generalization to human-directed empathy. *Anthrozoös*, **5**(3), 176–191.
3. Baarda, D. B. (1988) Schoolprestaties van kinderen van werkloze vaders. Thesis, University of Utrecht.
4. Bachman, R. W. (1975) Elementary school children perception of helpers and their characteristics. *Elementary School Guidance and Counselling*, **10**(2), 103–109.
5. Beck, A. and Katcher, A. H. (1984) A new look at pet-facilitated therapy. *Journal of the American Veterinary Medical Association*, **184**(4), 414–421.
6. Beck, A., Katcher, A. H. and Aoki, R. (1989) The influence of pets on the ability of children to recognize emotional signals in humans and animals. Paper presented at 5th International conference on the relationship between humans and animals. Monaco 1989.
7. Bekker, B. R. (1986) Adolescent pet owners vs. non-owners, friendship and loneliness. *Dissertation Abstracts International*, **47**, 1240.
8. Belsky, J. (1981) Early human experience, A family perspective. *Developmental Psychology*, **17**, 3–23.
9. Belsky, J. (1984) The determinants of parenting, A process model. *Child Development*, **55**, 83–96.
10. Bergesen, F. J. (1989) The effects of pet facilitated therapy on the self-esteem and socialization of primary school children. Paper presented at the 5th International conference on the relationship between humans and animals. Monaco 1989.
11. Blue, G. F. (1986) The value of pets in children's lives. *Childhood Education*, **63**, 84–90.
12. Bossard, J. H. S. (1944) The mental hygiene of owning a dog. *Mental Hygiene*, **28**, 408–413.
13. Brickel, C. M. (1982) Pet facilitated psychotherapy: A theoretical explanation via attention shifts. *Psychological Reports*, **50**, 71–74.
14. Bryant, B. K. (1985) The neighbourhood walk. A study of sources of support in middle childhood from the child's perspective. *Monographs of the Society for Research in Child Development*, **50** (serial no. 210).
15. Bryant, B. K. (1986) The relevance of family and neighbourhood animals to social–emotional development in middle childhood. Paper presented at the Delta Society International Conference, Boston, Massachusetts.
16. Bryant, B. K. (1990) The richness of the child–pet relationship: A consideration of both benefits and costs of pets to children. *Anthrozoös*, **3**(4), 253–261.
17. Bryant, B. K. and Whorley, P. (1989) Child–pet relationships under conditions of maternal unavailability. Paper presented at 5th International conference on the relationship between humans and animals. Monaco 1989.
18. Cain, A. O. (1985) Pets as family members. *Marriage and Family Review*, **8**, 5–10.
19. Cassel, J. (1976) The contribution of the social environment to host resistance. *American Journal of Epidemiology*, **104**, 107–123.
20. Cochran, M. and Brassard, J. (1979) Child development and personal social networks. *Child Development*, **50**, 601–616.
21. Cohen, S. and Wills, T. A. (1985) Stress, social support and the buffering hypothesis. *Psychological Bulletin*, **98**(2), 310–57.
22. Condoret, A. (1983) Speech and companion animals, experience with normal and disturbed nursery school children. In *New Perspectives in our Lives with Companion Animals*. Eds. A. H. Katcher and A. M. Beck. pp. 467–471. University of Pennsylvania Press, Pennsylvania.
23. Corson, S. A. and O'Leary Corson, E. O. (1987) Pet animals as social catalysts in geriatrics; an experiment in non-verbal communication therapy. In *Society, Stress and Disease, Old Age*. Ed. L. Levi. pp. 305–333. Oxford University Press, Oxford.
24. Covert, A. M., Whiren, A. P., Keith, J. and Nelson, C. (1985) Pets, early adolescents and families. *Marriage and Family Review*, **8**, 95–108.
25. Davis, J. H. (1987) Pre-adolescent self-concept development and pet ownership. *Anthrozoös*, **1**(2), 90–94.
26. Endenburg, N. (1991) Animals as companions; demographic, motivational and ethical aspects of companion animals ownership. Thesis, Amsterdam.
27. Furman, W. (1989) The development of children's social networks. In *Children's Social Networks and Social Support*. Ed. D. Belle. pp. 151–172. Wiley, New York.
28. Guttman, G., Predovic, M. and Zemanek, M. (1985) The influence of pet ownership in non-verbal communication and social competence in children.

Proceedings of the International Symposium on the Human–Pet Relationship. pp. 58–63. IEMT, Vienna.

29. Haggerty Davis, J., Gerace, L. and Summers, J. (1989) Pet-care management in child-rearing families. *Anthrozoös*, **2**(3), 189–193.

30. Harter, S. (1983) Developmental perspectives on the self-system. In *Handbook of Child Psychology, Socialization, Personality and Social Development.* Eds. E. M. Hetherington and P. H. Mussen. pp. 275–385. Wiley, New York.

31. Heath, T. D. and McKenry, P. C. (1989) Potential benefits of companion animals for self-care children. *Childhood Education*, **7**(4), 311–314.

32. Katcher, A. H. (1988) Touch, intimacy, nurturance: The biopsychology of human and animal companionship. Paper presented at the annual meeting of the Delta Society, Orlando, FL.

33. Levinson, B. M. (1969) *Pet-oriented Child Psychotherapy.* Charles C. Thomas, Springfield, IL.

34. Levinson, B. M. (1971) Household pets in training schools serving delinquent children. *Psychological Reports*, **28**, 475–481.

35. Levinson, B. M. (1978) Pets and personality development. *Psychological Reports*, **42**, 1031–1038.

36. Levinson, B. M. (1980) The child and his pet: A world of non-verbal communication. In *Ethology and Non-verbal Communication in Mental Health.* Eds. S. A. Corson, E. Corson and J. A. Alexander. pp. 63–83. Pergamon Press, Oxford.

37. MacDonald, A. (1981) The pet dog in the home. A study of interactions. In *Interrelations between People and Pets.* Ed. B. Fogle. pp. 195–206. Charles C. Thomas, Springfield, IL.

38. Melson, G. F. (1987) The role of pets in the development of children's nurturance. Paper presented to the annual meeting of the Delta Society. Vancouver, Canada.

39. Melson, G. F. (1988) Availability of and involvement with pets by children: Determinants and correlates. *Anthrozoös*, **2**(1), 45–52.

40. Melson, G. F. and Peet, S. H. (1988) Attachment to pets, empathy and self-concept in young children. Paper presented to the annual meeting of the Delta Society, Orlando, FL.

41. Messent. P. R. (1983) Social facilitation of contact with people by pet dogs. In *New Perspectives on our Lives with Companion Animals.* Eds. A. H. Katcher and A. M. Beck. pp. 45–67. University of Philadelphia Press, Philadelphia.

42. Messent, P. R. and Horsfield, S. (1985) Pet population and pet ownerbond. *Proceedings of the International Symposium on the Human–Pet Relationship.* pp. 9–17. IEMT, Vienna.

43. Mugford, R. A. and M'Comisky, J. G. M. (1975) Some recent work on the psychotherapeutic value of caged birds with old people. In *Pet Animals and Society.* Ed. R. S. Anderson. pp. 54–65. Charles C. Thomas, Springfield, IL.

44. Parry, G. and Shapiro, D. A. (1986) Social support and life events in working class women: Stress buffering or independent effects. *Archives of General Psychiatry*, **43**, 315–323.

45. Paul, E. S. (1992) Pets in childhood, individual variation in childhood pet ownership. PhD Thesis, University of Cambridge, England.

46. Poresky, R. H. and Hendrix, C. (1988) Developmental benefits of pets for young children. People, animals and the environment; exploring our interdependence. Paper presented at the Delta Society 7th Annual Conference.

47. Poresky, R. H. and Hendrix, C. (1989) Companion animal bonding, children's home environments and young children's social development. Paper presented at the Biennial Meeting of the Society for Research in Child Development, Kansas City, MI.

48. Poresky, R. H. and Hendrix, C. (1990) Differential effects of pet presence and pet-bonding on young children. *Psychological Reports*, **66**, 931–936.

49. Poresky, R. H., Hendrix, C., Mosier, J. E. and Samuelson, M. L. (1987) The companion animal bonding scale: Internal reliability and construct validity. *Psychological Reports*, **60**, 743–746.

50. Riksen-Walraven, J. M. A. (1978) *Stimulering van de Vroeg-kinderlijke Ontwikkeling, een Interventie Experiment.* Swets & Zeitlinger, Lisse.

51. Riksen-Walraven, J. M. A. (1983) Mogelijke oorzaken engevolgen van een (on)veilige eerste gehechtheidsrelatie, Een overzicht aan de hand van een model. *Kind en Adolescent*, **4**(1), 23–44.

52. Rispens, J., Goudena, P. P. and Groenendaal, J. H. A. (1994) *Preventie van Psychosociale Problemen bij Kinderen en Jeugdigen.* Bohn, Stafleu en van Loghum, Alphen a/d Rijn.

53. Robin, M., tenBensel, R. W., Quingly, J. S. and Anderson, R. K. (1983) Childhood pets and the psychosocial development of adolescence. In *New Perspectives in our Lives with Companion Animals.* Eds. A. H. Katcher and A. M. Beck. pp. 436–443. University of Pennsylvania Press, Philadelphia.

54. Ros, W. J. G. (1990) Sociale steun bij Kankerpatienten. Thesis, Amsterdam.

55. Rutter, M. (1990) Psychosocial resilience and protective mechanisms. In *Risk and Protective Factors in the Development of Psychopathology.* Eds. J. Rolf, A. S. Masten, D. Ciccetti, K. H. Nuechterlein

and S. Weintraub. pp. 181–215. Cambridge University Press, Cambridge.

56. Salomon, A. (1981) Animals and children, The role of the pet. *Canada's Mental Health*, **June**, 9–13.

57. Serpell, J. A. (1981) Childhood pets and their influence on adults' attitudes. *Psychological Reports*, **49**, 651–654.

58. Serpell, J. A. (1987) Pet keeping in non-western societies: Some popular misconceptions. *Anthrozoös* **1**(2), 166–174.

CHAPTER 3

The Role of Pets in Enhancing Human Well-being: Effects for Older People

LYNETTE A. HART

Introduction

The widespread ownership of pets among people of various ages and the effort and money spent on behalf of pets suggests that a majority of owners derive a significant benefit from their companionship. For families with growing children, pets can be part of the social support system[7] and provide opportunities to educate children and for them to experience nurturance.[46] For people in their later years, pet ownership may be more difficult than for younger people because of financial, physical, transportation and housing limitations or restrictions.

If definite benefits to older people arise from companionship with an animal, one could argue for encouraging pet adoption, just as exercise and nutritious diets are recommended for enhancing health. Such a recommendation would require having objective information concerning the specific circumstances where benefits are associated with pet ownership. Unfortunately, little is known specifically about which elderly people would benefit most or in which situations significant benefits would result. The purpose of this

chapter is to review studies that shed light on the role pets can play in enhancing the well-being of older people.

The first section of the chapter concerns healthy ageing and documents how the common preoccupation with elderly people in nursing homes is being supplanted with studies of healthy, older individuals who are responsible for their own well-being. The second section examines factors associated with pet ownership in older people. The next four sections of the chapter address particular effects of relationships with companion animals that are tailored to the life changes and common losses of elderly people. First, the socialising effects of animals, which may be important to elderly people who have lost friends and family members, especially if they lack children or employment to draw them into community activities. Second, the way in which pets may confer a role or identity on an individual. This may be important for someone whose life has revolved around professional, spousal and parental roles which may be lost as the person ages. Third, the stress reduction or buffering aspects of relationships with companion animals. These may assume special importance when key losses (such as death of a spouse) arise that jeopardise a person's well-being. Fourth, the motivating role of animals. This may help older people in providing nurturance to others and in participating in activities. The final section of the chapter focuses on some practical considerations regarding pet ownership for older people, such as obtaining housing where pets are permitted and arranging for various aspects of care.

Sustaining Well-being in Maturity

More than ever before, good health in the latter part of life is regarded as a result of taking healthy initiatives throughout life. A reversal of unhealthy practices (such as smoking) usually improves health. Even with cardiovascular crises that typically are handled with invasive surgery, a comprehensive array of major changes in lifestyle (including exercise, dietary changes, yoga or meditation), social support and community involvement can lead to some reversals of cardiovascular pathology.[52] In another extreme example involving AIDS patients, a programme of natural therapy combined with low dosages of drugs stimulated a reversal of the invasive disease from ARC (Aids Related Complex) to the less serious HIV infection in 6 of 19 patients.[32]

Evidence suggests that the ageing process itself can be retarded by a healthy lifestyle that addresses the psychological challenges arising in older years. People living as married couples have been shown to maintain significantly better psychological and physiological health when ageing than people living alone, especially men.[44] In addition, maintaining a regular daily routine is one of five key factors that is said to retard ageing.[9] However, much of life's familiar structure changes as one ages and healthy living requires an increasing initiative on the part of the older person.[16] For example, maintaining a regular daily routine can become difficult when a spouse dies. In a long-term study, Erikson *et al.*[16] found that elderly

people pointed to relationships with children and grandchildren as a source of strength that made their lives worthwhile. For some individuals pets may play a role somewhat analogous to that of children or grandchildren. Friedan[18] focused on the harmful stereotypes that hamper society's ability to draw from the wisdom of elderly people. Emphasising the importance of staying well, she argued for new methods of providing convenience and social support to older people and even went so far as to suggest that no more nursing homes for older people should be constructed.

The antiquated view of ageing as an inevitable decline with its ultimate prolonged disablement is simply not true in the western world where there are many opportunities for health and active involvement with life among people with a wide range of disabilities and diseases. Most of the research concerning the effects of interactions with pets for older people has been conducted in nursing homes or other institutional environments. Yet, the vast majority of elderly people live independently. In the USA, fewer than 5% of elderly people live in institutional settings and various estimates suggest that only between 10 and 40% of today's elderly people are expected to spend any time in a nursing home.[18] While it is true that elderly people may face certain challenges and stresses more often and sustaining the motivation to remain active and use time productively becomes increasingly challenging, they may also carry greater measures of wisdom and resources to sustain them than in their earlier years.

From lifelong longitudinal studies of people who are now elderly, Clausen[11] found that by adolescence some individuals exhibited a group of traits that strongly predicted and influenced their success throughout life. This cluster of traits was termed 'planful competence' and included dependability, intellectual involvement and self-confidence. Individuals with these traits were more able to cope with major challenging life transitions which for other individuals were overly daunting.

The Role of Pets in the Life Cycle

As proposed by Wilson and Netting,[74] the role of pets in people's lives can be viewed from the perspective of life course development. People's histories with pets are likely to influence their pattern of ownership, the benefits they derive from ownership, their perceptions of the pet's role and the degree to which the pet influences the person's sense of well-being. Having a close relationship with pets early in life would predict a close relationship later in life and a likelihood of benefiting from animal companionship. However, since longitudinal human studies on ageing have not monitored pet ownership, it is not possible to analyse lifelong patterns of pet ownership and relationships directly. However, questionnaires and surveys that assess personal histories of pet-keeping retrospectively have been administered to mature and elderly people.

Pet ownership patterns in childhood are key influences in pet ownership patterns as adults.[19] Among individuals aged 65–87 years, pet owners reported a past history of pet-keeping more frequently than did the non-pet owners.[34] In a study of adults, 88% of the pet owners had owned pets as children, as compared to only 28% of the non-pet owners,[36] and the strength of the relationship with pets was higher among pet owners who had experienced pets as children. People who have owned cats as children tend as adults to love cats and early experience with dogs predisposed a love of dogs.[35]

Studies focusing on various features of the relationship between dogs and humans were recently reviewed.[24] However, apart from the role of personal history in influencing pet selection throughout life, surprisingly few studies have sought to compare relationships with cats versus dogs. The information is not available to know in what circumstances a cat might be a more appropriate companion for an older person than a dog. Presumably, the activity level of some breeds of dogs may be aversive to an older person who has physical disabilities, is frail, or is bedridden much of the time. A recent study of men with AIDS indicated that cats were well suited for the needs of individuals with compromised health.[8] While less interactive than dogs, cats offer many aspects of the social interactions sought by lonely people.[45]

Some pet owners feel closer to their animals than to family members, as was illustrated when people drew diagrams representing their family members and 38% of dog owners placed the dog closer to themselves than any other family member.[4] While it might appear paradoxical, pet ownership is highest among families with young children, whereas relationship strength is, on average, highest in small families or among individuals who live alone.[2,36,59]

Close relationships with pets in pet-owning families has been significantly related to family adaptability, presumably through family members experiencing negotiations on the roles, rules and responsibilities of having a pet.[14] A strong relationship with pets was also related to family cohesion, as measured by emotional bonding, boundaries, time use, decision making, interests, recreations and coalitions. This study of family functioning suggests that a close relationship with a pet may be a broad indicator of healthy human or family relationships.

In one study, elderly women aged 65–75 years who had a better relationship with their pets were more likely to be closely attached to their spouses and to be happy.[53] Both high income and a strong relationship appeared to be prerequisites for a positive effect of pets on morale. Pet owners with limited income had low scores on general happiness, perhaps partially reflecting the financial obligations of pet keeping.

Simply owning a pet does not assure it a significant role. Negative results were reported in a study of elderly women, where the strength of the relationship with their pets was unrelated to levels of depression.[48] An exploratory study of war veterans with a mean age of 63 years reported an association of pet ownership with improved morale and health,[56] but with a full sample, no differences were observed between pet owners and non-owners.[57] These negative findings illustrate the importance of identifying the types of individuals or circumstances in which animals may contribute a benefit.

Some studies have documented healthier self-ratings among adult pet owners than non-owners and one study reported higher achievement scores among pet owners than non-owners.[10] The owners valued the reciprocal relationships with the animals that were characterised by unconditional acceptance, love, affection, laughter, play and protection. The responsibility of pet ownership was mentioned as a disadvantage and was also the main stated reason for non-ownership of pets.

When men and women over 65 years of age provided self-ratings on a standardised test, pet owners described themselves with more favourable adjectives, such as nurturance, independence, optimism.[34] Male non-owners scored higher than male owners and all females, on arrogance and hostility. Consistent with other studies, pet owners more often than non-owners had kept pets in past years. In interviews with elderly men and women living alone and receiving home delivery of meals, the pet owners scored lower on loneliness than the non-owners.[55]

Socialising Effects of Companion Animals

The need for social contact and support is often not met for older individuals, who may have lost many friends due to death. Also, they generally no longer have employment to structure their daily schedules and provide social interactions. Health or financial constraints may curtail activities that formerly kept them socially involved. However, older individuals can remain socially engaged in various ways, through special interests such as a companion animal, by participating in community or religious organizations, or by assisting family members with child care.

Even people who have an animal companion require human companionship. An animal companion can greatly facilitate establishing friends and much work over the past decade has focused on the socialising effects of companion animals.[15,29,58] A classic study in 1975 reported the 'social lubricant' and 'ice-

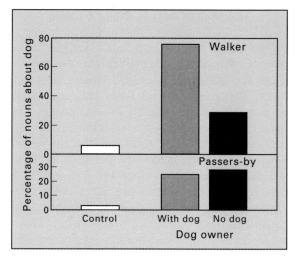

FIG. 3.1: Percentage of nouns concerning people or animals that referred to a dog, as spoken by the walker or the passers-by greeted on the walk.[58]

breaker' functions of pet birds for men and women aged 75–81 years.[49] Although the participants had a high attrition rate, the group with a pet bird appeared to show social and psychological improvements.

In a recent study of people aged 65–78 years walking their dogs in their neighbourhood, the dog was a major focus of conversations with passers-by, as shown in Fig. 3.1.[58] While walking, non-owners spoke very little about animals, whereas dog owners spoke about their dogs even when walking without them. Dog owners' conversations focused on the present or future (Fig. 3.2), whereas non-owners' conversations during

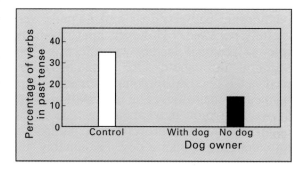

FIG. 3.2: Percentage of verbs in the past tense in conversations of a walker and passers-by, as a function of dog ownership and the presence of the walker's dog.[58]

walks featured past events. In another study, even a small animal such as a rabbit or turtle, readily attracted unfamiliar passers-by of all ages to converse with a woman sitting in a park.[29] Conversations focused on the animal, sometimes involving a personal anecdote about an animal from the passer-by.

Unfamiliar passers-by have been shown to respond with friendly interest, smiles and conversations more often to a person using a wheelchair who is accompanied by an assistance dog than when the person is without their dog.[15] Thus, we know from observations of human behaviour in a wide range of circumstances that a companion animal readily elicits friendly responses, even from unfamiliar passers-by.

In a study of elderly persons receiving home assistance,[75] all had a close relationship with their pets and most reported confiding in the pet more easily than in other people. Touching pets made 74% feel better. Once given access to a veterinarian, study participants made frequent calls, which appeared to be 'more related to a need for social interaction than to actual problems'.

Various studies conducted in institutional environments have used an experimental design to examine the effects of introducing an animal on the social behaviour of people. When a dog or a photographic stimulus was presented to elderly female patients in two wards, patients showed increased social interactions amongst themselves and with the staff when the dog was present, as judged by an independent observer and in ratings by ward nurses.[27] In another visiting programme at a residential home, residents interacting with puppies and their handlers showed improvements in their social interaction, psychosocial function, life satisfaction, mental function, level of depression, social competence and psychological well-being in comparison with the control group.[17] Nursing home patients with Alzheimer's disease showed improved social interactions amongst themselves and with staff and increased calmness, when provided with weekly interactive sessions with Golden Retrievers.[6] The presence of a dog also increased social behaviours in another study for patients with Alzheimer's disease, but placing the dog permanently in the facility was no better for the patients than the temporary visits.[37] A study of elderly women patients in long-term care provided them with a weekly one hour leisure activity and a one hour pet therapy session with a rabbit for six weeks.[33] In the first sessions, more positive social responses occurred during the pet therapy session than the leisure sessions. By the sixth week, the pet therapy session maintained its strong effect and although the leisure session had increased its effect, more laughing occurred overall during the pet therapy than during the leisure sessions.

If pets facilitate socialisation of people in various settings, it could be assumed that this at least partially results from interacting with the pet. Miller *et al.*[47] examined differences among 230 independently living pet owners over 50 years of age. Those who reported either some degree of inconvenience or some degree of uplift from their pets were termed the 'interacters', as compared with those who reported neither inconvenience nor uplift from their pets. The interacters were slightly younger, more educated and in better health than the non-interacters. The interacters were significantly more satisfied with life and had higher positive expectations (Fig. 3.3). Twenty-five percent of the study participants were men. For the men, any uplift from pets was associated with worries in the areas of social interactions, time and money, suggesting that pets were playing a compensatory social role. Uplift from pets was reported by women who had leisure time and a lack of psychological pressure.

For older individuals whose social involvement is limited, companion animals themselves can be an accessible source of social and tactile contact. Observations of nursing home residents in two facilities during a dog's visit showed that 85–93% of residents groomed or touched the dog on average 15–25 times per person.[50] In-home observations of families' interactions with dogs indicate that dogs adjust the frequencies of their

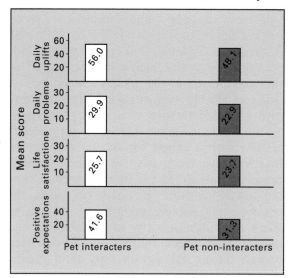

FIG. 3.3: Mean scores for pet interacters and pet non-interacters on positive expectations, life satisfaction, daily problems and daily uplift.[47]

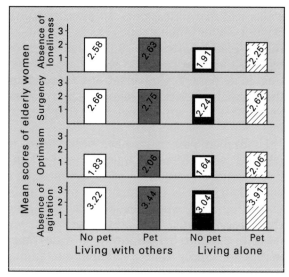

FIG. 3.4: Morale scores of elderly women. The effects of living alone or with other people and with or without pets.[21]

interactions with family members in response to the person's behaviour and interest.[68]

In a study of elderly women, pets made a difference in well-being for those living alone, but no difference for those living with others.[21] Compared with non-owners, pet owners living alone had significantly higher morale on four of the six psychological scales, including absence of agitation, optimism, surgency (a measure of active initiative for activity) and absence of loneliness (Fig. 3.4). Pet owners living alone actually scored higher than pet owners living with others on absence of agitation, but this was not mentioned nor tested statistically by the author.

For some older individuals, a companion animal provides essential social contact. In one study of elderly dog owners who lived alone, 75% of males and 67% of females said their dog was their only friend.[54] They reported talking to their dogs as if they were human, felt that their dogs fulfilled a need for companionship and that their relationship with the dogs was as strong as with humans. The dogs gave them something to do with their time and fulfilled their need to nurture. Women especially appreciated the loyalty of dogs.

The Influence of Pets on Personal Identity

A feeling of uselessness can be an immediate consequence following retirement.[22] Pets instantly confer roles (e.g. cat lover or dog owner) on those who appreciate animals. These roles are identities shared with others and they echo across past, present and future involvement with animals. When emerging themes were drawn from interviews and observations of six elderly women, the primary theme was that the pet was an integral part of the person's identity.[61] It was also shown that pet-owning could enhance or detract from social relationships and that the pet was a 'significant other' in the daily lives of the subjects.

Assuming an identity as someone who loves animals can establish a link with others who have a similar identity. An ethnographic study at three geriatric facilities documented that pet visitation produced a family atmosphere symbolising and re-creating domesticity.[60] Residents readily shared personal information about their families, their health, their roommates, their religious beliefs, their job experiences and the homes they had given up. These unintended social effects were characterised by reminiscing, intimacy and bonding with the volunteers who had brought the animals. The pets were found to facilitate interaction between people rather than being the main focus of interaction itself. Perhaps volunteers are motivated to bring pets into facilities by the ability of their pets to create a safe, enjoyable and intimate context with others who also love pets, much as in therapeutic horseback riding where the presence of horses creates a joyful occasion for the people who are gathered.[23]

The Role of Pets in Stress Reduction

A concept consistent with many studies is that a companion animal can reduce transient or significant stress, buffering the effect of the stress on the person. Allen *et al.*[3] documents how subjects exposed to a transient stressor such as performing a challenging arithmetic problem, showed a reduction in stress in the presence of their dog than when in the presence of a close friend. In another study, participants given the task of reading aloud experienced anxiety above baseline, in contrast with either reading quietly or interacting with a friendly unfamiliar dog, which resulted in reduced anxiety.[73] These studies are discussed in detail in the next chapter and although not focusing on older people, there is no reason to expect that similar effects will not occur in all age groups.

Individuals endure a profound ongoing stress when they lose a spouse, particularly if the spouse was virtually the sole confidant, and such a loss is increasingly likely to occur as people grow older. With the combined stress of losing a spouse and the subsequent social isolation, a person could be vulnerable to depression. In such a circumstance, pet owners reported significantly less depression than non-owners.[20] Among pet owners who had lost a spouse and had few confidants, those who had a strong relationship with their pet experienced less depression than those whose relationship was less strong. Related findings of more psychogenic symptoms and higher drug use among non-owners than pet owners were reported in a study of

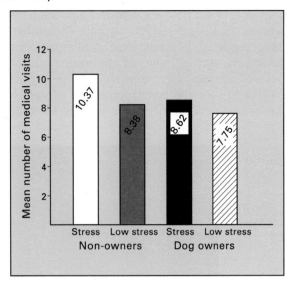

FIG. 3.5: Mean number of medical visits as a function of dog ownership and stress.[66]

people who had been widowed within the previous 3 years.[1]

Siegel's[65,66] study of medical visits by elderly people provided further evidence for the stress buffering hypothesis. When compared with non-owners, pet owners made fewer medical visits over the course of a year. A more pronounced effect was found when stressful life events during the 6 months before the study were considered. As shown in Fig. 3.5, non-owners experiencing stressful life events increased their medical contacts, whereas dog owners with similar stressful events did not show an increase. Dog owners reported spending 1.5 hours per day talking to their dogs and felt more secure than non-owners. Owners believed that they spent more time with their dogs than did other pet owners, that they felt closer to their pets than other owners and that there were more positive than negative effects of having pets. Siegel concluded that dog ownership influences coping ability for dealing with losses.

The Role of Pets in Facilitating Healthy Activities

As discussed earlier, when people age it becomes increasingly important that they choose a lifestyle which will help them to remain healthy.[16] Older people themselves have reported psychological challenges presented by ageing.[5] One of the major contributions made by animals is providing motivation for the constructive use of time.[43] An animal can motivate a person to keep going, get up in the morning and follow a routine. Virtually all dog owners report that their dogs enjoy walks.[62] Dogs also provide motivation for a wide range of interactive behaviours.

Melson's[45] studies have emphasised the importance of children being able to nurture

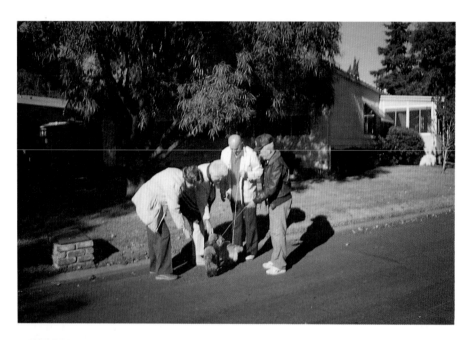

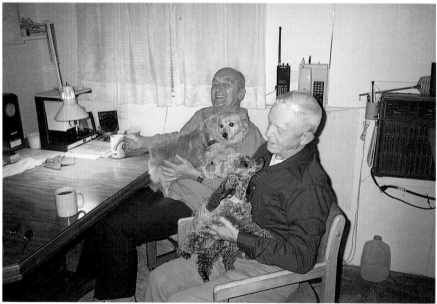

FIG. 3.6: (top) A typical daily walk for two men and their dogs.
(bottom) The aftermath of the walk.

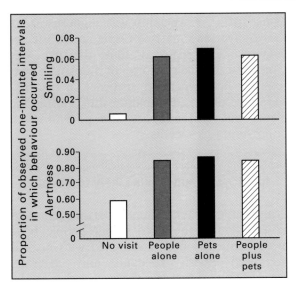

F<small>IG</small>. 3.7: Proportion of observed 1 minute intervals in which alertness or smiling occurred under various visiting conditions.[28]

animals, especially for the youngest or only child who lacks the opportunity to care for a younger sibling. As people become older, they may once again come to have few opportunities for nurturing; this is particularly true for men. Animals are effective in stimulating nurturing from many men and women. Among older pet owners in one study, 84% of men and 75% of women often played with their pets.[69]

Perhaps the most widely known aspect of human–animal interactions is pet visits to elderly people in nursing homes. Volunteers with animals have probably visited facilities in most communities in the USA and many programmes occur in other countries. Although various studies have investigated the effects of such visits for patients or staff, the role of animals in motivating the volunteers to participate in this activity has received little mention. A study of participants in volunteer training workshops for animal-assisted therapy documented that for these individuals, their animals acted as social catalysts, making their interactions with other humans easier and more enjoyable.[70] Such studies are important because while animals are frequently credited with helping nursing home residents, the benefits may accrue from the human as well

as the animal visitor. As shown in Fig. 3.7, Hendy's[28] study found that human visitors alone were as effective as pets alone or human visitors with pets, in eliciting smiling and alertness responses from patients. Human visitors influenced the nursing home residents more than the pets, but the pets may be essential because of their ability to motivate the visitors to make, increase or extend their visits to the nursing home.

Corson and Corson[13] described how animals acted as socialising catalysts with patients and staff and thus improved the overall morale of the institution and created a community out of detached individuals. In other studies with visiting animals, the increased motivation of the staff translated into improved morale, patient–staff communication and, presumably, enhanced care for patients.[6]

In a longitudinal study of elderly persons, pet attitudes, ownership and mutual activities with pets significantly predicted health and morale for some people.[39] Serpell's longitudinal study of lifestyle changes following pet adoption, although not focusing on older people, found that people adopting dogs sharply increased their time walking.[63,64] Siegel's study of elderly people also documented that dog owners spent 1.4 hours per day outside with the dog.[65,66] Exercise is now seen as essential for human health. It plays a central role in avoiding hip fracture[12,40] and is an essential component of cardiovascular medical programmes.[52] Dogs seem to provide the motivation for adults of various ages to participate in regular outdoor exercise which will contribute to increased health.

Practical Considerations

Although many studies have demonstrated benefits from pets, not everyone chooses, or is able, to own one. Over half of elderly, former pet owners in one study reported that they did not desire a pet.[75] In another study of older people, 39% currently preferred non-involvement with pets.[72] Respondent characteristics associated with non-involvement included age, poor visual acuity and limited physical mobility or use of arms. Having insufficient indoor and outdoor space was characteristic of the residential settings among people preferring non-involvement. Virtually all these respondents reported considerable involvement with animals earlier in their lives, but some had shifted to preferring a more indirect and passive involvement. A study of participation by institutional residents in various activities suggested that if assistance with pets was more readily available, the extent of participation would reflect both the personal characteristics of the people and the features of the housing environment.[42]

Older people often reduce the size of their homes and in doing so they make choices that may support or detract from their sustaining an involved lifestyle. For people who choose to live in ground floor accommodation, outdoor access is relatively easy, which would facilitate dog or cat ownership.[26] However, a widespread problem is that in rented accommodation pets are often not permitted and living on upper floors may reduce the ease of pet ownership. In the USA, older people living in State or Federally assisted housing have some protected rights to own pets, while those living in privately owned housing must rely on the willingness of the property owner. A recent study in the UK[31] found that the 'no pet' policy of many nursing homes for older people caused stress and anguish to older pet owners. Some people even missed hospital appointments because they feared referral to a home where no animals were allowed. More worrying was the lack of written policy concerning pets in many establishments. Regulations preventing pet ownership are usually drawn up to prevent potential problems. However, older people living in assisted housing in California were found to be extremely responsible pet owners and the problems with property damage and personal injury that were anticipated when pets were first introduced, did not occur.[25]

In a recent survey of 1595 people aged 60 years and over, living in Illinois, USA, 32.7% owned pets.[67] Ownership was highest among the younger and married residents. Of the pet owners, 86% reported that the pet was important in their choice of housing. Reasons for pet ownership, in order of priority, were love of pets, companionship, getting the owner out of the house and providing an opportunity to socialise.

Identifying Individuals Likely to Benefit

Programmes where animals have been used in an attempt to benefit older people have most frequently been conducted with institutionalised elderly residents and generally have not identified the characteristics of the individuals who showed improvement. In one study with volunteers and dogs visiting twice weekly for 12 weeks, the elderly residents reported less depression, anxiety, anger, fatigue and confusion, compared to the control residents.[71] Further analyses showed that individuals with strong positive past experiences and current attitudes toward pet animals accounted for the improvement, whereas individuals with less positive attitudes and experiences had not shown a significant improvement.

Among people living independently, those living alone appeared less likely to own pets.[41] As contributing factors to non-ownership, they had lower incomes and lived in multi-home apartments. Some individuals who had formerly kept pets later decided not to have them. Impaired health, advanced age and more confined housing were some reasons given in a longitudinal study for giving up pet-keeping.[38] Among those who managed to keep pets through the third year of this study, involvement with the pet and the pet's sleeping location were effective predictors of morale and self-rated physical health.

Many critical variables influence a person's choice of pet, including the past events and previous attitudes to and relationships with pets. Current health status, the housing situation, whether one lives alone, the amount of time to be spent with a pet and the socioeconomic status are other relevant variables.[74]

In interviews with older men and women in Arizona, the type of housing, close relationships with pets in childhood and health status accounted for 24% of the variance in predicting pet ownership.[51]

Older people living independently may have difficulties in keeping up with the various responsibilities of pet care, including grooming, veterinary care and shopping for food. Others are concerned about what would happen to a pet if they should die or need hospitalisation. Volunteer or paid help where needed, would make it more feasible for some people to keep pets longer. Extensive efforts focus on bringing visiting pets into institutions, yet few organised programmes provide support for pet-keeping to older people who live independently. Some imaginative programmes do exist. In Scotland, there is a charity which provides emergency care for a pet, in the homes of volunteers, should an elderly owner be unable to care for the animal. In the USA there is a programme which matches older people who would like a pet with older pets in need of a home. However, these pet adoption schemes must have sufficient support and follow-up to ensure that the adoption is mutually beneficial.

From the work discussed in this chapter, it seems clear that at least for some older individuals, a companion animal contributes to enhanced socialisation, an identity, stress reduction and motivation. Therefore a future goal for the various governmental and non-governmental organisations which assist older people should be to provide support for those people who desire to own or have contact with a pet.

Acknowledgements—A generous contribution from Kal Kan Foods, Inc. made this review possible. Bonnie Mader provided the photographs.

References

1. Akiyama, H., Holtzman, J. M. and Britz, W. E. (1986–87) Pet ownership and health status during bereavement. *Omega*, **17**, 187–193.
2. Albert, A. and Bulcroft, K. (1988) Pets, families and the life course. *Journal of Marriage and the Family*, **50**, 543–552.
3. Allen, K. M., Blascovich, J., Tomaka, J. and Kelsey, R. M. (1991) Presence of human friends and pet dogs as moderators of autonomic responses to stress in women. *Journal of Personality and Social Psychology*, **61**, 582–589.
4. Barker, S. B. and Barker, R. T. (1988) The human–canine bond: Closer than family ties? *Journal of Mental Health Counseling*, **10**, 46–56.
5. Berman, P. L. (1989) *The Courage to Grow Old.* Ballantine Books, New York.
6. Beyersdorfer, P. S. and Birkenhauer, D. M. (1990) The therapeutic use of pets on an Alzheimer's unit. *American Journal of Alzheimer's Care and Related Disorders and Research*, **5**, 13–17.
7. Bryant, B. (1985) The neighborhood walk: Sources of support in middle childhood. *Monographs of the Society for Research in Child Development*, **50** (3, Serial No. 210).
8. Castelli, P., Hart, L. A. and Zasloff, R. The comforting role of cat companionship for persons with AIDS diagnoses. *Submitted.*
9. Chopra, D. (1993) *Ageless Body, Timeless Mind.* Harmony Books, New York.
10. Chouinard, B. E. (1991) A comparison of personality variables of pet owners and non-pet owners. PhD Thesis, Pepperdine University.
11. Clausen, J. A. (1993) *American Lives: Looking Back at the Children of the Great Depression.* Free Press, New York.
12. Cooper, C., Barker, D. J. P. and Wickham, C. (1988) Physical activity, muscle strength and calcium intake in fracture of the proximal femur in Britain. *British Medical Journal*, **297**, 1443–1446.
13. Corson, S. A. and Corson, E. O'L. (1981) Companion animals as bonding catalysts in geriatric institutions. In *Interrelations Between People and Pets.* Ed. F. Fogle. pp. 146–174. Charles C. Thomas, Springfield, IL.
14. Cox, R. P. (1993) The human/animal bond as a correlate of family functioning. *Clinical Nursing Research*, **2**, 224–231.
15. Eddy, J., Hart, L. A. and Boltz, R. P. (1988) The effects of service dogs on social acknowledgments of people in wheelchairs. *Journal of Psychology*, **122**, 39–45.
16. Erikson, E. H., Erikson, J. M. and Kivnick, H. Q. (1986) *Vital Involvement in Old Age.* W. W. Norton & Company, New York.
17. Francis, G., Turner, J. T. and Johnson, S. B. (1985) Domestic animal visitation as therapy with adult home residents. *International Journal of Nursing Studies*, **22**, 201–206.

18. Friedan, B. (1993) *The Fountain Of Age*. Simon & Schuster, New York.

19. Gage, M. G. (1988) *Family Careers and Companion Animal Experience: A Study of Anticipatory Socialization*. CENSHARE, University of Minnesota, Minneapolis.

20. Garrity, T. F., Stallones, L., Marx, M. B. and Johnson, T. P. (1989) Pet ownership and attachment as supportive factors in the health of the elderly. *Anthrozoos*, **3**, 35–44.

21. Goldmeier, J. (1986) Pets or people: Another research note. *The Gerontologist*, **26**, 203–206.

22. Gubrium, J. F. and Lynott, R. J. (1983) Rethinking life satisfaction. *Human Organization*, **42**, 30–38.

23. Hart, L. (1992) Therapeutic riding: Assessing human versus horse effects. *Anthrozoos*, **5**, 138–139.

24. Hart, L. A. (1995) Dogs as human companions: A review of the relationship. In *The Domestic Dog*. Ed. J. Serpell. Cambridge University Press (in press).

25. Hart, L. A. and Mader, B. (1986) The successful introduction of pets into California public housing for the elderly. *California Veterinarian*, **40(5)**, 17–21.

26. Hart, L. A., Fox, S. and Rogers, J. (1992) Acceptance of dogs and cats in mobile home parks. *Canine Practice*, **17(1)**, 24–28.

27. Haughie, E., Milne, D. and Elliott, V. (1992) An evaluation of companion pets with elderly psychiatric patients. *Behavioural Psychotherapy*, **20**, 367–372.

28. Hendy, H. M. (1987) Effects of pet and/or people visits on nursing home residents. *International Journal of Aging and Human Development*, **25**, 279–291.

29. Hunt, S. J., Hart, L. A. and Gomulkiewicz, R. (1992) Role of small animals in social interactions between strangers. *Journal of Social Psychology*, **132**, 245–256.

30. Johnson, M. A. (1988) Variables associated with friendship in an adult population. *The Journal of Social Psychology*, **129**, 379–390.

31. Joseph Rowntree Foundation (1993) Joseph Rowntree Foundation Social Care Research Findings No. 44.

32. Kaiser, J. D. (1994) *Immune Power*. St. Martin's, New York.

33. Kalfon, E. (1991) Pets make a difference in long-term care. *Perspectives*, **15(4)**, 3–6.

34. Kidd, A. H. and Feldmann, B. M. (1981) Pet ownership and self-perceptions of older people *Psychological Reports*, **48**, 867–875.

35. Kidd, A. H. and Kidd, R. M. (1980) Personality characteristics and preferences in pet ownership. *Psychological Reports*, **46**, 939–949.

36. Kidd, A. H. and Kidd, R. M. (1989) Factors in adults' attitudes toward pets. *Psychological Reports*, **65**, 903–910.

37. Kongable, L. G., Buckwalter, K. C. and Stolley, J. M. (1989) The effects of pet therapy on the social behavior of institutionalized Alzheimer's clients. *Archives of Psychiatric Nursing*, **3**, 191–198.

38. Lago, D. H., Connell, C. M. and Knight, B. (1985) The effects of animal companionship on older persons living at home. *Proceedings of the International Symposium on the Occasion of the 80th Birthday of Nobel Prize Winner Professor Dr Konrad Lorenz*, pp. 328–340. Institute for Interdisciplinary Research on the Human–Pet Relationship, Austrian Academy of Sciences, Vienna, Austria.

39. Lago, D., Delaney, M., Miller, M. and Grill, C. (1989) Companion animals, attitudes toward pets and health outcomes among the elderly: a long-term follow-up. *Anthrozoos*, **3**, 25–34.

40. Lau, E., Donnan, S., Barker, D. J. P. and Cooper, C. (1988) Physical activity and calcium intake in fracture of the proximal femur in Hong Kong. *British Medical Journal*, **297**, 1441–1443.

41. Lawton, M. P., Moss, M. and Moles, E. (1984) Pet ownership: A research note. *Gerontologist*, **24**, 208–210.

42. Lemke, S. and Moos, R. H. (1989) Personal and environmental determinants of activity involvement among elderly residents of congregate facilities. *Journal of Gerontology: Social Sciences*, **44**, S139–148.

43. Levinson, B. M. (1969) Pets and old age. *Mental Hygiene*, **53**, 364–368.

44. Lynch, J. J. (1977) *The Broken Heart: The Medical Consequences of Loneliness*. Basic Books, New York.

45. Mahalski, P. A., Jones, R. and Maxwell, G. M. (1988) The value of cat ownership to elderly women living alone. *International Journal of Aging and Human Development*, **27**, 249–260.

46. Melson, G. F. (1988) Availability of and involvement with pets by children: Determinants and correlates. *Anthrozoos*, **2**, 45–52.

47. Miller, D., Staats, S. and Partlo, C. (1992) Discriminating positive and negative aspects of pet interaction: Sex differences in the older population. *Social Indicators Research*, **27**, 363–374.

48. Miller, M. and Lago, D. (1990) The well-being of older women: The importance of pet and human relations. *Anthrozoos*, **3**, 245–251.

49. Mugford, R. A. and M'Comisky, J. G. (1975) Some recent work on the psychotherapeutic value of caged birds with old people. In *Pet Animals and Society*. Ed. R. S. Anderson. pp. 54–65. Baillere-Tindall, London.

50. Neer, C. A., Dorn, C. R. and Grayson, I. (1987)

Dog interaction with persons receiving institutional geriatric care. *Journal of the American Veterinary Medical Association*, **191**, 300–304.

51. Netting, F. E., Wilson, C. C. and Fruge, C. (1988) Pet ownership and nonownership among elderly in Arizona. *Anthrozoos*, **2**, 125–132.
52. Ornish, D. (1990) *Doctor Dean Ornish's Program for Reversing Heart Disease.* Ballantine Books, New York.
53. Ory, M. G. and Goldberg, E. L. (1983) Companion animals and elderly women. In *New Perspectives on our Lives with Companion Animals*. Eds. A. H. Katcher and A. M. Beck. pp. 303–317. University of Pennsylvania Press, Philadelphia.
54. Peretti, P. O. (1990) Elderly–animal friendship bonds. *Social Behavior and Personality*, **18**, 151–156.
55. Ramnath, M. S. (1988) Pet ownership and loneliness in the elderly who live alone and receive mobile meals. MSN Thesis, Medical College of Ohio at Toledo.
56. Robb, S. S. (1983) Health status correlates of pet-human association in a health impaired population. In *New Perspectives on our Lives with Companion Animals.* Eds. A. H. Katcher and A. M. Beck. pp. 318–327. University of Pennsylvania Press, Philadelphia.
57. Robb, S. S. and Stegman, C. E. (1983) Companion animals and elderly people: A challenge for evaluators of social support. *Gerontologist*, **23**, 277–282.
58. Rogers, J., Hart, L. A. and Boltz, R. P. (1993) The role of pet dogs in casual conversations of elderly adults. *The Journal of Social Psychology*, **133**, 265–277.
59. Salmon, P. W. and Salmon, I. M. (1983) Who owns who? Psychological research into the human–pet bond in Australia. In *New Perspectives on our Lives with Companion Animals*. Eds. A. H. Katcher and A. M. Beck. pp. 244–265. University of Pennsylvania Press, Philadelphia.
60. Savishinsky, J. S. (1986) The human impact of a pet therapy program in three geriatric facilities. *Central Issues in Anthropology*, **6(2)**, 31–41.
61. Schulman, K. R. (1989) The phenomenology of elderly pet ownership: Partners in survival. EdD, Syracuse University.
62. Serpell, J. A. (1981) The personality of the dog and its influence on the pet–owner bond. In *New Perspectives on our Lives with Companion Animals*. Eds. A. H. Katcher and A. M. Beck.

pp. 57–63. University of Pennsylvania Press, Philadelphia.
63. Serpell, J. A. (1990) Evidence for long term effects of pet ownership on human health. In *Pets, Benefits and Practice*. Ed. I. H. Burger. Waltham Symposium 20, pp. 1–7. BVA Publications, London.
64. Serpell, J. (1991) Beneficial effects of pet owenrship on some aspects of human health and behavior. *Journal of the Royal Society of Medicine*, **84**, 717–720.
65. Siegel, J. M. (1990) Stressful life events and use of physician services among the elderly: The moderating role of pet ownership. *Journal of Personality and Social Psychology*, **58**, 1081–1086.
66. Siegel, J. M. (1993) Companion animals: In sickness and in health. *Journal of Social Issues*, **49**, 157–167.
67. Smith, D. W. E., Seibert, C. S., Jackson, F. W. and Snell, J. (1992) Pet ownership by elderly people: Two new issues. *International Journal of Ageing and Human Development*, **34**, 175–184.
68. Smith, S. L. (1983) Interactions between pet dog and family members: An ethological study. In *New Perspectives on our Lives with Companion Animals*, Eds. A. H. Katcher and A. M. Beck. pp. 29–36. University of Pennsylvania Press, Philadelphia.
69. Stallones, L., Marx, M. B., Garrity, T. F. and Johnson, T. P. (1988) Attachment to companion animals among older pet owners. *Anthrozoos*, **2**, 118–124.
70. Stein, M. A. and Bergin, B. M. The human/companion animal bond enhances motivation for voluntarism. Unpublished manuscript.
71. Struckus, J. E. (1989) The use of pet-facilitated therapy in the treatment of depression: A behavioral conceptualization of treatment effect. PhD Thesis, University of Massachusetts.
72. Verderber, S. (1991) Elderly persons' appraisal of animals in the residential environment. *Anthrozoos*, **4**, 164–173.
73. Wilson, C. C. (1991) The influence of a pet as an anxiolytic intervention. *Journal of Nervous and Mental Disease*, **179**, 482–489.
74. Wilson, C. C. and Netting, F. E. (1987) New directions: Challenges for human–animal bond research and the elderly. *Journal of Applied Gerontology*, **6**, 189–200.
75. Wilson, C. C., Netting, F. E. and New, J. C. (1985) Pet ownership characteristics of community-based elderly participants in a pet placement program. *California Veterinarian*, **39(3)**, 26–28.

CHAPTER 4

The Role of Pets in Enhancing Human Well-being: Physiological Effects

ERIKA FRIEDMANN

Introduction

People believe that pets are important. This is evident in popular culture where a dog is considered to be 'man's best friend'. In fact a multitude of articles appear in the non-professional press documenting the extraordinary abilities of some pets to assist, sense danger for, protect and even save their owners. While many of these claims are spurious or questionable, the public continues to look for confirmation of the popular and logical belief that pets are somehow good for people. There are also many anecdotal reports of the benefits individuals have experienced as a result of becoming pet owners. New pet owners may become calmer, more relaxed, more willing to venture out into the world and begin interacting with people. These anecdotal reports provide confirmation that at least some people believe that pets provide concrete measurable benefits. However these reports alone do not provide sufficient evidence to substantiate this claim and the

question remains, how do people benefit from their pets? There are many perspectives for addressing this problem. The idea of physiological health benefits that might traverse the life cycle is particularly attractive. Current theories of health provide a framework to conceptualise potential physiological benefits for people from their pets.

In the latter half of the 20th century, members of the health professions have come to recognise how dramatically health depends upon interpersonal aspects of an individual's life. The influence of these factors on psychological disorders was recognised before it was realised that they had an effect on a broader range of diseases. Social, psychological and physiological factors are now widely recognised as factors influencing the development and progression of many chronic or stress related diseases. Within holistic models of health, an individual's social and psychological states are thought to determine the impact of both external and internal insults or challenges on health. Social, psychological

Erika Friedmann

and even spiritual factors can act either to promote health by moderating or serving as buffers in the relationship between stressors and stress related diseases, or to promote disease by enhancing or promoting pathological responses to stressors.[4] Within the last two decades, recognition of the role of psychosocial factors in health has expanded tremendously. The diverse group of conditions which involve psychosocial components includes, but is not limited to: asthma, cancer, colds, colitis, coronary heart disease, eczema, headaches, hypertension, impotence and ulcers.[22] The idea that social and psychological factors can mediate the long term effects of stress, led to the investigation of their roles in the development and progression of chronic diseases which are the most common causes of death in modern society.[22] It also provided a rationale for examining the possibility that we obtain health benefits from our pets.

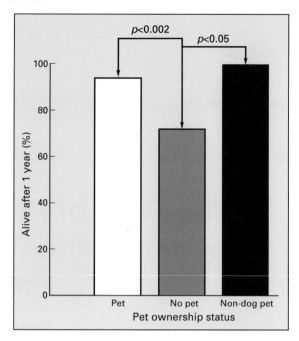

FIG. 4.1: Comparison of 1 year survival rates after admission to a coronary care unit between pet owners, non-owners and owners of a 'non-dog' pet.[15]

Evidence for Health Benefits from Pets

Pets and Cardiovascular Health

The chronic nature of cardiovascular disease, and its status as a leading cause of death in western societies, led to a study on the social, psychological and physiological factors in coronary heart disease (CHD) and their relevance to patients' survival. The importance of social support for cardiovascular health had already been established.[23] Pet ownership was included as one source of social support expected to improve survival of patients hospitalised for coronary heart disease. In this first study of the relationship between pet ownership and cardiovascular health,[15] pet owners were more likely to be alive one year after discharge from a coronary care unit than non-owners. Only 5.7% of the 53 pet owners compared with 28.2% of the 39 patients who did not own pets died within one year of hospitalisation (Fig. 4.1). The possibility that dog owners were generally more healthy than other patients because they had to walk their dogs was

considered. In order to control for the potential effects of better health being required to care for a dog, dog owners were removed from the data set. The relative survival rates of patients who owned pets other than dogs and those who did not own any pets were then compared. The percentage of people who owned pets other than dogs who were alive one year after admission to a coronary care unit was still greater than people who did not own pets. Thus, even when dog owners were eliminated, survival was more frequent for pet owners than non-owners. While pet ownership was related to survival, there were several questions about the relationship that remained unanswered. One of the possible explanations for this finding was that pet owners were initially healthier than non-owners. If that were true, the relationship between pet ownership and survival would just have been an expression of the relationship between disease severity and mortality. A third analysis permitted examination of the independent roles of pet ownership and disease severity in survival. The

RESULTS OF DISCRIMINANT ANALYSES			
Variable	**% of Total Variation Explained**	**% Variation Added**	**Significance of Addition**
Severity	21.0	21.0	.001
Severity + pet ownership*	23.5	2.5	.004
Severity + pet ownership + age**	24.9	0.6	NS
Severity +age**	21.9	0.9	.014
* variance added and significance tested are for pet ownership. ** variance added and significance tested are for age. NS Not significant at p < .05.			

FIG. 4.2: Results of discriminant analyses used to examine the interactive and independent effects of physiological severity index and pet ownership on one year survival of patients admitted to a coronary care unit.[15]

severity of each patient's illness was estimated with an index, which included severity of the current disease (heart attack or severe angina pectoris), previous heart attacks and presence of congestive heart failure or left ventricular hypertrophy. Discriminant analysis was then used to examine how well the severity index predicted survival status after one year and the independent contribution of pet ownership to survival. As expected, the most important predictor of survival of the CHD patients was disease severity, which predicted 21% of the variance. Pet ownership made a significant contribution beyond the predictive value of illness severity alone (Fig. 4.2). Thus pet ownership made a contribution to survival, independently of the severity of the disease. An additional question asked was whether pet ownership was a substitute for or the equivalent of other forms of social support. However, the data showed that the relationship of pet ownership to survival was independent of other sources of social support. Being married or living with others were not significant predictors of survival. The sample was small and precluded addressing questions about what types of pets might prove to be most beneficial. The potential of pet ownership to promote health was documented, but

the direct mechanism of this benefit was not determined.

A recent large scale epidemiological study has provided evidence that pet ownership may protect people from developing coronary heart disease or slow its progression. It addressed the differences between pet owners and non-owners on physiological variables associated with increased risk of developing coronary heart disease, confronting some of the same issues evaluated in the study of survival by patients with coronary heart disease. Anderson *et al.*[3] examined standard cardiovascular risk factors among 5741 people attending a screening clinic in Melbourne, Australia. Risk factors refer to physiological, behavioural, or environmental elements that are associated with an increased likelihood of developing a specific disease. In order to ascertain that the individuals in this sample were representative of the population, the risk factors for coronary heart disease were compared with the risk factors found in the Australian National Heart Foundation's random survey. This indicated that the sample resembled the general population of Australia with respect to the risk factors.

The risk factors present in the pet owners and non-owners were then compared. When

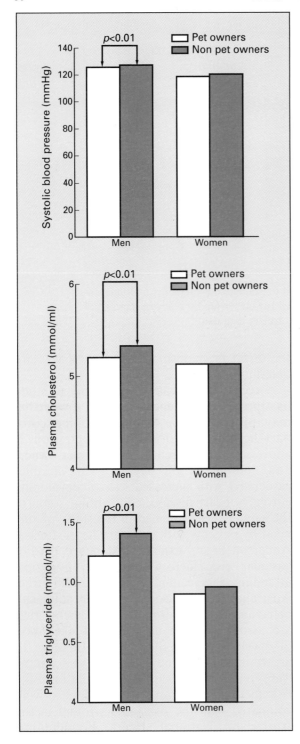

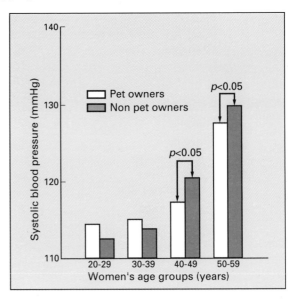

FIG. 4.4: Comparison between pet owners' and non-owners' average systolic blood pressure for women aged 20–59 years according to age.[3]

FIG. 4.3: Comparison between pet owners' and non-owners' average (top) systolic blood pressure, (middle) plasma cholesterol and (bottom) plasma triglyceride levels for men and women aged 20–59 years.[3]

the 784 pet owners aged 20–59 years were compared with the 4957 non-owners, the pet owners had lower systolic blood pressures and plasma triglycerides than the non-owners. When men and women were examined separately, male pet owners had significantly lower systolic blood pressure, plasma cholesterol and plasma triglyceride levels than the non-owners (Fig. 4.3). For women, the only differences between pet owners and non-owners were among those who were most vulnerable to coronary heart disease, namely those who were over 40 years old. Among women over 40, systolic blood pressure was lower for the pet owners than the non-owners (Fig. 4.4). Neither body mass index, an indicator of physical fitness, nor diastolic blood pressures differed between pet owners and non-owners.

Lifestyle factors which increase the risk of cardiovascular disease were also compared. Pet owners were more likely to be drinkers, to eat take away meals and to consume meat more than seven times per week, but were also more likely to be physically active. Thus pet owners did not behave in a consistently more healthy manner than non-owners. Differences in healthy behaviours could not be the sole cause of the differences in risk factors between pet owners and non-owners.

The social and economic status of pet owners and the non-owners were also compared but no differences in either socio-economic status or income estimates were found. Thus the risk factors associated with pet ownership were not reflections of differences in known risk factors among the different socio-economic groups.

Risk factors in dog owners and owners of other pets were compared to address the possibility that the differences in risk factors for pet owners were due to the exercise which occurs while walking a dog. There were no differences in blood pressure, cholesterol or triglyceride levels between dog owners and owners of other pets, although dog owners did have higher body mass indices than non-owners. For the general population, a higher body mass index usually indicates higher levels of body fat. This suggests that dog owners were likely to be more obese than owners of other pets, although this difference did not generate significant differences in the other risk factors measured.

Pets and General Health

Many studies use cross-sectional survey techniques to compare the health status of pet owners and non-owners. Cross-sectional studies allow the simultaneous assessment of many variables at one point in time. Although such studies are useful for identifying relationships among variables, one must be careful not to infer cause and effect from data of this type. The two studies discussed above, support the concept that pets might be associated with decreased risk and slower progression of coronary heart disease. Other reports suggest that pet ownership is associated with superior adjustment to bereavement,[1,7,19] use of physicians[42] and emotional health.[19] However, surveys of some populations have concluded that pet ownership was not related to health status.[36,38,43]

In contrast to cross-sectional studies, longitudinal studies provide evidence of causation

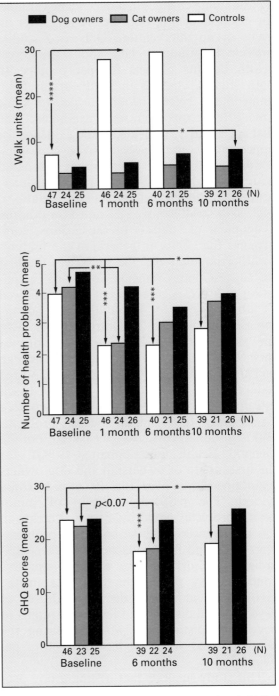

FIG. 4.5: Average (top) number of walk units, (middle) number of minor health problems, and (bottom) psychological distress as measured by scores on the General Health Questionnaire (GHQ) for individuals who acquired dogs and cats, and members of the control group at baseline and after 6 and 10 months. *$p < 0.05$, **$p < 0.01$, ***$p < 0.001$, ****$p \ll 0.001$.

by examining changes in a dependent variable, for example health, both before and after an event or an intervention. Only two studies provide longitudinal data about the direct health benefits of pets for pet owners. In both studies, changes in health status from immediately before owning a pet to some time after acquisition were examined. The first such study,[35] provided some evidence for improvements in the social and psychological condition of people given birds, compared with those who received a plant or no intervention. Although methodological limitations, such as a small sample size and non-random assignment of subjects to the groups, compromise the ability to generalise the findings to other populations,[6] the study was the first to suggest improvements following acquisition of a pet. A more recent study followed 71 adult subjects for 10 months after acquiring a cat or dog and 26 control subjects over the same period.[41] Dog owners improved their physical exercise habits through increased walking (Fig. 4.5) and reported reduced fear of crime and improved self esteem. Both dog and cat owners reported significantly fewer minor health problems and emotional concerns (measured on the General Health Questionnaire, GHQ), for the first month of ownership and dog owners maintained this over the 10 month study period. The reduced reporting of minor health problems could indicate a decrease in the occurrences of these common problems (e.g. colds and flu, headaches, hay fever and indigestion), or that the owners were less concerned by them. The decreases in the GHQ score indicate a decreased degree of psychological distress and fewer symptoms of psychiatric disturbances after acquiring the pet compared with the baseline before pet ownership.

This study suggests that getting a dog provided some long term health benefits. These benefits could have been the result of increased physical activity associated with walking the animal. In fact, the lack of such long term benefits for cat owners supports this possibility. However, it is important to note that people chose to be pet owners; pets were not randomly assigned. The evidence does however provide additional support for direct health benefits from pet ownership.

A Mechanism for Physiological Effects from Pets

While the studies discussed provide considerable evidence for the physiological benefits of pets, important questions remain unanswered. The first is an issue of causation. Was the pet a cause of the improved health or decreased risk, or was there a common factor which caused both pet ownership and health benefits? The second is an issue of mechanism. How could pets decrease the development and progression of coronary heart disease and how could this effect be documented?

Based upon a theoretical perspective, three mechanisms for the health benefits from pets for cardiovascular patients and for the population as a whole have been suggested.[14,25] The basic idea was that when people get upset, they have a stress response often called the **fight or flight response**. This is a coordinated mobilisation of the body's systems which includes activation of the sympathetic nervous system, leading to increases in blood pressure and heart and respiratory rate, as well as hormonal changes which prepare the individual to fight or flee from some foe. This response is adaptive if the person is going to fight or flee. The body uses the changes to maximise the physical exertion required to fight or flee and the physiological levels return to normal after the burst of activity. If the individual does not perform a burst of physical activity, the built up hormones, high blood pressure and other factors continue and there is no quick return to normal levels. While the preparation gradually dissipates, an additional burden is placed on the body until this occurs. Frequent repetition or sustained periods of this mobilisation response can cause damage to the cardiovascular system.

Common stress reduction techniques such as relaxation, positive mental imagery and yoga, rely on helping a person to be less reactive to stressors, to redefine stressors to be less intense, or to remove the built up stress hormones quickly. It was reasoned that these stress reduction mechanisms might also apply to pets. Pets could help people either avoid a stress response entirely, by altering a situation that would otherwise be stressful or by mitigating the stress response by decreasing the impact of the stressor. Furthermore, pets could help individuals remove the built up stress hormones from their bodies more rapidly, by encouraging their owners to exercise.

Thus, it has been hypothesised that pets can decrease anxiety and sympathetic nervous system arousal by providing a pleasant external focus for attention, promoting feelings of safety and providing a source of contact comfort.[14] They can decrease loneliness and depression by providing companionship, promoting an interesting and varied lifestyle and providing an impetus for nurturing. Certain types of pet could help improve physical fitness by providing a stimulus for exercise. Pets therefore have the potential to moderate the development of stress related diseases such as coronary heart disease and hypertension. The range of benefits that owners might derive from their pets may not pertain only to pet owners; one could speculate that anyone, not just pet owners, could benefit from the presence of friendly animals. However, benefits may be dependent on the extent of involvement with the animal (for example non-owners might not have an opportunity to nurture an animal) and the type of animal (for example fish do not provide a source of contact comfort).

The focus of the remainder of this chapter will be the anti-arousal effects of friendly animals. Research was developed to test the hypothesis that pets can have direct effects on cardiovascular health by decreasing or preventing the physiological or psychological manifestations of stress including anxiety and elevation of blood pressure. Research on the stress reducing effects of pets has focused on two related areas: the effects of being in the presence of animals and the effects of interaction with animals.

Effects of the Presence of a Friendly Animal

A friendly animal may cause short term anti-anxiety and anti-arousal effects. The lower a person's level of anxiety, the less the sympathetic nervous system is activated and thus the smaller the response to a given stressor. If a scene or situation is perceived as less anxiety-inducing there will be a less extreme physiological response to it. Even an unknown animal can have a positive impact on psychological perceptions and on physiological indicators of stress such as blood pressure and heart rate (HR). A series of studies has documented the anti-arousal effects of friendly animals. Initial studies documented the impact of animals on people's perceptions of scenes and of the people in them. Further studies examined reductions in physiological arousal when a friendly animal was present in a stressful situation and have begun to investigate factors that determine who will benefit most from the presence of a friendly animal.

People have long thought that the presence of an animal induces changes in perceptions of situations and the people in them. Artists, publicists and advertisers have used animals effectively to influence our moods and perceptions. Research findings support the positive effects of animals on people's moods and perceptions. The first study to address how the presence of a friendly animal affects people's perceptions, addressed the effect of the presence of the researcher's dog. In a complex design, 10 dog owners and 10 non-owners were exposed to psychological testing in two settings. Each subject was tested in a psychological laboratory, which was considered to be a high stress situation, and in their own home, which was considered to be a low stress situation.[40] For each subject, the researcher was accompanied by her dog to one of these two sessions. The subjects indicated significantly lower anxiety on a psychological checklist and behaved significantly less anxiously in the high stress environment when the dog accompanied the researcher than when no dog was present (Fig. 4.6). There were no differences in the responses of the dog owners and non-owners. Of particular interest was the finding that the subjects paid more attention to the researcher's dog in the high than in the low stress situation. This suggests that the relaxing external focus of attention or feelings of safety pro-

vided by a friendly animal might be particularly important in stressful situations.

The effect of an animal's presence on people's perceptions of situations was confirmed in a related study.[31] Instead of placing people in situations and comparing their perceptions with and without animals present, this study employed pictures of scenes with and without animals present. A series of scenes, based on the Thematic Apperception Test card model, with one or two people in a natural environment were printed in two forms. One form contained a scene with people and one or more animals (Fig. 4.7) present and the second form contained the same scene without animals. Subjects were asked to rate both the scenes and the people in them by referring to contrasting adjective pairs in a check list. Adjective pairs used to rate the scenes included: pleasant–unpleasant; humorous–serious; friendly–hostile; safe–dangerous; relaxed–tense; constructive–destructive. Adjective pairs used to rate the people in the scenes included: healthy–unhealthy; confident–worried; curious–disinterested; happy–sad; comfortable–uncomfortable; gentle–rough; friendly–unfriendly; harmless–dangerous. This test is now called the Animal Thematic Apperception Test (ATAT). The ATAT scenes and the people in them were perceived as significantly more friendly, less threatening and happier when animals were included in these scenes than when animals were absent.

These studies show that the presence of an animal can influence an individual's psychological perceptions. Animals had a positive effect on individuals' perceptions of both their personal environments and of pictures of people and their environments. It is an individual's perceptions of the nature of a situation and the people in it that determine the magnitude of the stress response. The more threatening a situation, the larger the physiological arousal that occurs. Thus, these findings were consistent with the hypothesis that the presence of an animal would decrease physiological arousal, although that hypothesis had to be addressed more directly.

The next step was to investigate whether the presence of animals could act directly as

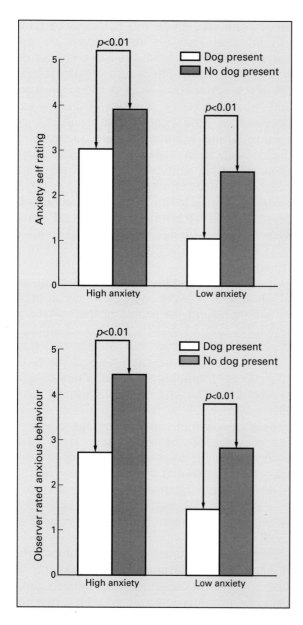

FIG. 4.6: Effect of the presence of a dog on subjects' self rated anxiety (top) and observer rated anxious behaviour (bottom) in high anxiety and low anxiety situations.[40]

an anti-arousal agent and modify the physiological responses occurring during stressful activities. The development of automated oscillometric blood pressure devices allowed the non-invasive study of cardiovascular arousal during speech. A striking association between speaking and rapid, significant elevations in blood pressure and heart rate was demonstrated in several studies (Fig. 4.8).[32,44] This response occurred consistently in populations ranging in age from young children to elderly individuals, coronary heart disease patients, hypertensive and normotensive individuals, in men and women of various races and socio-economic groups and in environments as varied as clinics, classrooms and work places. The magnitude of the increase was moderated by a number of

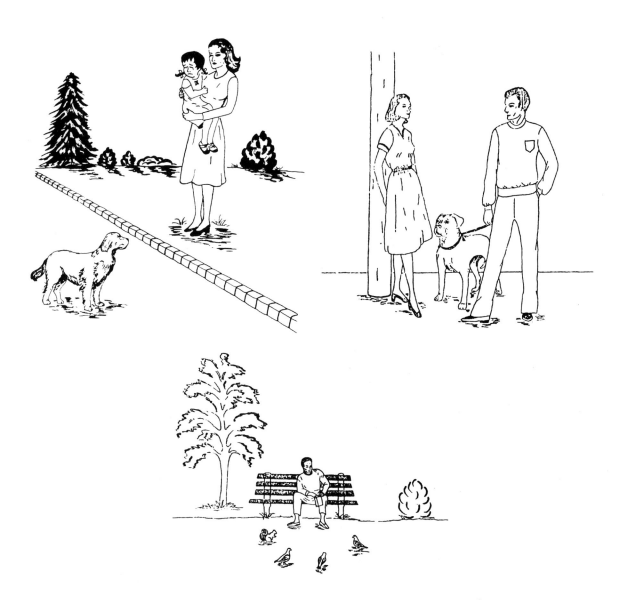

FIG. 4.7: The road, post and bench scenes with animals present used to develop the Animal Thematic Apperception Test. The identical scenes without the animals present were also used in the development of the tool.[12,30]

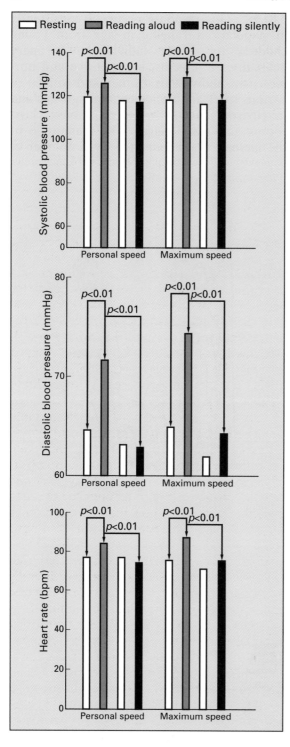

FIG. 4.8: Average systolic blood pressure (top), diastolic blood pressure (middle) and heart rate (bottom) while resting, reading aloud and reading silently at both maximum and personal speeds.[16]

factors including the rate of speech, status of the interviewer, audience size, affective content and baseline blood pressure. The increases in blood pressure were greater when speaking rapidly than slowly, when speaking to a higher than a lower status individual, when speaking in front of a group than an individual, when the topic had greater affective content than when the content was more neutral and when the subjects were hypertensive than when they were normotensive. It was also noted that the cardiovascular response during reading aloud was similar to the response during talking. Thus, reading aloud became a standard way of providing uniformity and minimising the affective content of the speech and provided a method for investigating the effects of social and behavioural factors on the magnitude of the cardiovascular response.

The effects of an animal's presence on cardiovascular changes occurring during speech were examined in 38 children, aged 9–15 years.[17] Children's blood pressures and heart rates were measured while they rested silently and read aloud both with and without an unfamiliar but friendly dog accompanying the researcher. The order of the series (dog accompanying the researcher or researcher only) was randomly determined and the effects on the children's blood pressures of both the presence of the animal and the order of the series, were examined. Average mean arterial (MAP), systolic (SBP) and diastolic (DBP) blood pressures during the entire experiment were lower for the children who had the dog present during the beginning of the experiment than for those who had the dog present for the second half of the experiment. Blood pressures were consistently significantly higher (DBP: 8 mmHg, SBP: 6.1 mmHg) while reading aloud than while resting but the presence of the dog attenuated the blood pressure response (Fig. 4.9). The presence of the dog in the first series was also associated with lower blood pressures during the entire procedure. The attitude of the subjects toward dogs or toward pets in general was not addressed and differences between children whose families

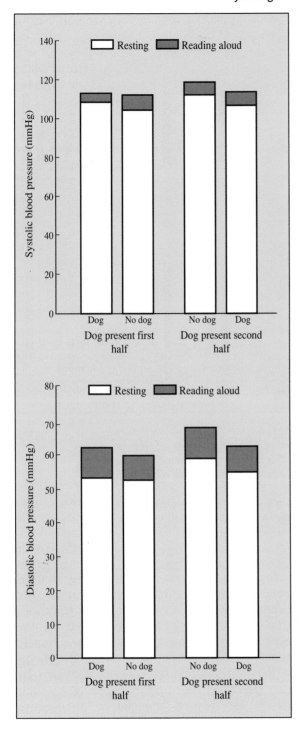

FIG. 4.9: Average systolic (top) and diastolic (bottom) blood pressures while resting silently and reading aloud with and without a friendly dog present, comparing subjects with the dog present for the first half and second half of the protocol.[17]

had pets and those who did not were not investigated. However, this study provided the first direct evidence that the presence of animals could moderate stress responses.

A similar study was subsequently conducted among college students. In this study the coronary prone behaviour pattern, Type A was also assessed. The National Heart Lung and Blood Institute have recognised that Type A behaviour pattern (TABP) is an independent risk factor for coronary heart disease.[37] Individuals who are Type A are characterised by hard driving, ambitious, competitive and time urgent behaviour while those who are Type B tend to exhibit a relaxed more serene style of behaviour.[11,39] Since the 1970s, studies examining the physiological basis for the association between coronary prone or Type A behaviour and coronary heart disease have focused on the acute change in a cardiovascular variable (i.e. blood pressure or heart rate) that is attributed to a behavioural stimulus.[9,33] In CHD patients and Type A individuals, chronic heightened cardiovascular responses to various types of stressors have been implicated as a causative factor in the progression of and mortality from hypertension[8,10] and coronary heart disease.[28,29] In the study of the effect of a dog's presence on 193 Type A and Type B college students, the presence of a dog caused significant moderation of heart rate, but not blood pressure, responses among both Type A and Type B individuals.[18,30]

While the preceding studies showed that the presence of an unfamiliar but friendly dog can influence an individual's stress responses to reading aloud, the ability of a person's own dog or a dog's effect on other types of stressor was not addressed. A study of the cardiovascular responses of dog owning college students to the presence of their own dogs during two types of cognitive stress yielded somewhat different results.[21] Neither blood pressure nor heart rate responses during mental arithmetic and psychological assessment were different for the 16 college students accompanied by their dogs during the experimental protocol than for the 16 dog owners who were unaccompanied. One

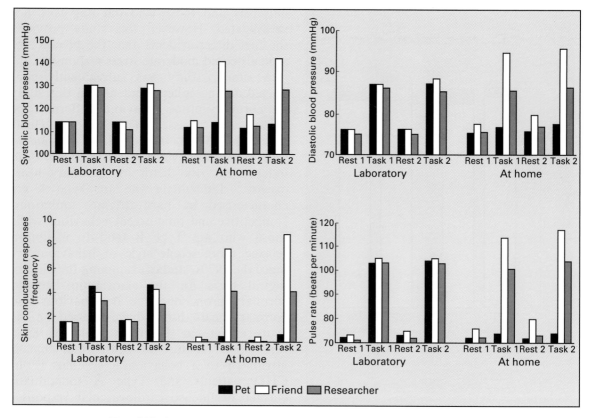

FIG. 4.10: Average systolic blood pressure, diastolic blood pressure, skin conductance and pulse (heart) rate during alternate periods of resting (Rest 1 & 2) and stressful tasks (Tasks 1 & 2 of mental arithmetic). The subjects (all female) were split into 3 groups and tested in their own home with either their pet present, a female friend present or only the researcher present. The same subjects were also tested in a laboratory environment with only the researcher present, but data were subdivided into the home testing subject groups for comparative purposes.

could speculate that having to control their pets in the laboratory situation might be stressful for the dog owners. Attempting to complete a cognitive task while controlling one's dog might be particularly difficult. It is also possible that the benefits of an animal's presence depend on the type of stressor. Perhaps the presence of an animal is less effective at reducing the responses to cognitive stressors than to interpersonal stressors. This question has not been directly addressed, although in other settings, the presence of an animal has been associated with decreased cardiovascular responses to a cognitive stressor.

A further study using mental arithmetic as a cognitive stressor addressed the role of social support in modifying the cardiovascular response.[2] Women's cardiovascular responses to a stressful task were evaluated in the presence of the subject's own dog or a female friend. The intent was to compare the effects of the non-judgmental support provided by their pets with the support provided by their friends for women engaged in a cognitive task. Consistent with previous research on the cardiovascular response to reading aloud,[16,17,32] in the laboratory all physiological measures rose significantly during mental arithmetic. In the home setting cardiovascular responses were significantly greater

ADJECTIVE PAIRS USED TO ASSESS MOOD OF THE SCENE

Friendly–hostile
Humorous–serious
Romantic–unromantic*
Pleasant–unpleasant
Relaxed–tense*
Constructive–destructive*
Cooperative–uncooperative
Safe–dangerous*

*Semantic differential items worded in opposite direction to avoid scoring bias.[12]

FIG. 4.11: Adjective pairs included in the scale (FSCENE) used to assess the mood of the scene.

ADJECTIVE PAIRS USED TO ASSESS PERCEPTIONS OF THE WOMAN AS NURTURING

Generous–stingy*
Harmless–dangerous
Sympathetic–unsympathetic*
Gentle–rough
Friendly–unfriendly*
Trustworthy–untrustworthy

*Semantic differential items worded in opposite direction to avoid scoring bias.[12]

FIG. 4.12: Adjective pairs included in the scale (FNURT) used to assess perceptions of the woman in the scenes as nurturing.

when the female friend was present than when only the researcher was present and were lower when the dog was present (Fig. 4.10). These data show that the presence of the woman's dog moderated her stress response more than the presence of a supportive friend. The authors concluded that the non-judgmental aspect of the support afforded by the pet was responsible for decreasing the stress response.

The magnitude of the effect of an animal's presence on the stress response may be determined by a combination of factors. The type and familiarity of the situation, type of stressor and relationship with or attitudes to the animal could all have an influence. In Allen *et al.*'s study[2] the positive effects of the dog's presence were found in the home,

rather than a laboratory setting. This situation is very different from the one reported by Grossberg *et al.*[21] where the student's pet came into the unfamiliar laboratory situation and no beneficial effect was recorded. Based upon limited studies, the presence of an animal may be less useful for moderating the effects of cognitive rather than interpersonal stressors. The combination of an unfamiliar laboratory situation and a cognitive stressor may be so stressful for the dog owner that it negates the positive, stress reducing effect of the pet's presence. It appears that pet ownership *per se* is not necessary for an individual to receive physiological benefits from the presence of a pet. However, pet owners may benefit more than non-owners in specific situations. Among pet owners, the closeness of the relationship with the pet is likely to be one determinant of the magnitude of the benefits. However this issue has not been systematically addressed.

Individuals may not benefit equally from the presence of pets. It would be expected that individuals who perceive animals more positively would receive greater cardiovascular benefits from an animal's presence than those who perceive animals less positively. This supposition was addressed using the physiological data from college students[18,30] in conjunction with information about their attitudes toward animals obtained with the ATAT described above.[12] The effects of attitudes toward dogs on cardiovascular responses during reading aloud were assessed when a friendly but unfamiliar dog was present.[13] Attitudes toward dogs were assessed using individual's perceptions of a scene containing a dog (Fig. 4.7) and the woman in it. Two separate ATAT scales were used. Perceptions of the scene as having a positive mood were assessed using the FSCENE scale (Fig. 4.11) and of the woman in the scene as nurturing were assessed using the FNURT scale (Fig. 4.12). Attitudes towards dogs as assessed by both the FSCENE scale and the FNURT scale were related to cardiovascular responses. The blood pressure responses when reading aloud with a dog present were significantly lower for those with a more

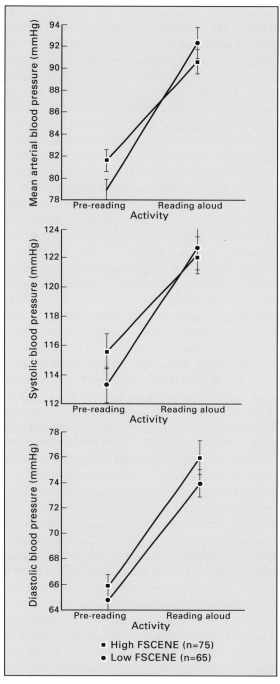

FIG. 4.13: Average mean arterial (top), systolic (middle) and diastolic (bottom) blood pressures while resting and reading aloud with a dog present according to the subjects' perceptions of the road scene including the dog. High scores on the FSCENE scale are indicative of more positive perceptions of the road scene with the dog in it. Error bars are ± standard error of the mean.[13]

positive attitude toward dogs (i.e. in subjects who had scored higher on the FSCENE or FNURT scales) than those with a more negative attitude toward dogs (Figs 4.13 and 4.14). The presence of the dog moderated the physiological response of those who had a more positive attitude toward dogs. The results of this study were the first to confirm that an individual's attitude towards animals was related to the cardiovascular benefit they received from them, independently of their pet ownership status. Thus, attitudes about specific pets may be related both to the cardiovascular benefit individuals receive from the presence of the animal and to whether people choose to keep pets.

The great majority of the research documenting the direct effect of an animal's presence on health concerns involves dogs. Indeed, most laboratory research on the physiological effects of animals has been limited to dogs. Dogs are particularly convenient to use because they are easily available and they willingly assume the desired roles in research protocols. However, there is no reason to expect that benefits occur only for dogs. Other species should have similar effects, but the usefulness of a species for promoting health might depend, at least partially, on an individual's attitude toward the species and the individual animal in particular.

To date, information about the physiological effects of other animals is limited and mainly concerns the effects of looking at an aquarium. Watching fish in aquaria can lead to decreases in both blood pressure and anxiety. One study reported reductions in the blood pressures of patients with hypertension, that were similar to those reported for relaxation therapy, biofeedback or transcendental meditation.[26] The researchers wondered whether it was the fish in the aquarium or perhaps the focus of attention on a distractor, that led to these decreases. In order to confirm that the effects were due to the fish and not the pleasant bubbling water and plants, two comparisons were conducted. The decreases in blood pressure which occurred while looking at fish swimming were compared with those which

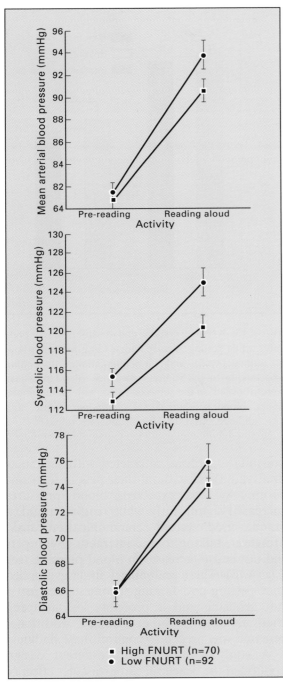

FIG. 4.14: Average mean arterial (top), systolic (middle) and diastolic (bottom) blood pressures while resting and reading aloud with a dog present according to the subjects' perceptions of the woman in the road scene including the dog. High scores on the FNURT scale are indicative of perceptions of the woman in the road scene as more nurturing. Error bars are ± standard error of the mean.[13]

occurred while looking at an identical tank without fish and while looking at a poster of a pleasant scene. The decreases continued for a longer period when looking at fish swimming than when looking at either of the other soothing stimuli. Similarly, the cardiovascular response to speech was diminished after watching the fish swimming compared with the beginning of the session. The decreases in resting blood pressure and the responses to speech were most pronounced in those subjects whose initial blood pressures were highest.

In a further study, the benefit of observing a tank of fish immediately before a stressful experience was evaluated.[27] For 42 dental patients, watching a fish swim in an aquarium before dental surgery proved to be an effective means of increasing patient compliance and of decreasing perceptions of pain during the dental procedure. Furthermore, the effect of watching fish was approximately equivalent to the effect of hypnosis. Since looking at fish is an excellent and easy method to achieve relaxation, it may well be an effective way of reducing anxiety in heart disease patients. Based upon the differences in psychological responses, one would expect that the cardiovascular stress responses of those who watched a fish tank before surgery would also be reduced compared with those who did not watch a fish tank.

The studies of dogs and fish demonstrate that the presence of friendly animals can cause a decrease in physiological and psychological responses to moderately severe stressors, which may be influenced by an individual's perceptions of the animals. However, different mechanisms may be responsible for the effects from dogs or fish. It has been suggested that the distraction of looking at the constant activities of the 'natural world' of the fish tank encourages people to look outside themselves. This is similar to the relaxation induced by various forms of meditation or hypnosis. The fish tank, with its infinite variety and movement provides a focus for even untrained individuals who are directed to contemplate it. This idea contrasts dramatically with studies of the presence of the dog.[13,17,18,30] The dog was not a focus of attention, in fact it was out of the subject's direct line of sight. The subject's attention was not directed at the dog and the dog was not moving in an interesting or attractive way, it was lying calmly at the researchers' feet. In this situation, just the presence of the dog, without it directly receiving attention, was sufficient to moderate cardiovascular responses. Previous personal or even vicarious pleasurable experiences with dogs may be sufficient for the presence of a dog to induce memories which are pleasurable and calming. Fish might have similar effects, but this has not been tested.

Effects of Interacting with a Friendly Animal

A second group of studies has focused on the effects of interacting with pets on blood pressure and on mood. Again, there was no reason to believe that the benefits of interacting with animals would be limited to the owners of the animals. Initial studies consisted of observing interactions between people and their animals in order to learn, more systematically, how people interact with their pets and with other friendly animals. The two most frequent types of interactions with pets were touching and talking to the animal. These observations led to the question of whether contact comfort obtained from touching a friendly animal provides a physiologically calming influence.

Researchers began to investigate whether touching a pet provided physiological benefits to its owner. Shortly after beginning this study, it became apparent that in a mildly stressful situation, people do not just touch their pets; people talk to them at the same time.[24] It was almost impossible for pet owners to touch their dogs or cats without talking to them at the same time. Thus the first study was revised to study the effects of interacting with rather than just touching the pet. The physiological effects of interacting with a pet were compared to those of interacting with other people. Blood pressures of 35 pet owners, recruited from a veterinary clinic waiting room, were measured while they rested without their pets in a private

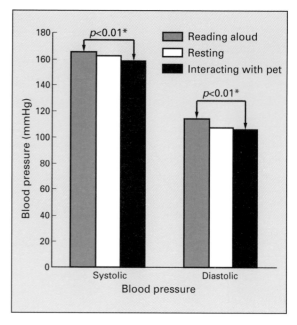

FIG. 4.15: Average systolic and diastolic blood pressures while resting silently and reading aloud without an animal present and while interacting with, petting and talking to the subject's own pet. Blood pressures were recorded on the subjects' calves with an automatic digital blood pressure device. *Non parametric rank difference test used for significance values.[24]

consultation room, interacted with their pets and read aloud without their pets in the same room. As was expected, blood pressures increased significantly while reading aloud, a standardised verbal communication task. However, talking to and interacting with pets did not cause increases in blood pressure (see Fig. 4.15). These preliminary findings implied that petting and talking to one's own pet is not arousing and is probably less arousing than talking to other people. Additional research was needed to confirm these findings.

A study with a slightly different design confirmed the beneficial cardiovascular effect of petting one's own pet.[5] The effects of petting one's own dog, without talking to it, were compared with the effects of petting an unfamiliar dog and with the effect of reading silently. Blood pressures and heart rate were recorded for 9 minutes in all three conditions and the order of the conditions was varied. Systolic and diastolic blood pressures decreased significantly from the first to the final assessment while the 24 dog owners petted their own dogs but not the unfamiliar dog; heart rate was not affected by petting (see Fig. 4.16). Since blood pressures continued to fall in the last period, the duration of the calming effect of petting requires further investigation. The beneficial effect of petting was limited to the owners' dogs. When subjects began interacting with their own pets there was a 'greeting response' during which the highest blood pressures were recorded. This may have been related to stress associated with having to control the dog in the laboratory environment. If the initial measurements were not included, the differences between the two types of dog may not be significant. This study improved on the previous study by altering the order of the activities, but the effect of petting the dogs was not compared with the effects of interacting with people or of any other stressor.

A more recent study confirmed that interaction with a friendly but unfamiliar dog can reduce the physiological and psychological consequences of stress for dog owners and non-owners.[46,47] Blood pressures and heart rate were measured during 10 minute activities: reading aloud, reading quietly and interacting with a friendly but unfamiliar pet. The order of the activities was varied. Anxiety was measured while the subject was resting between treatments. In this study of 92 self selected undergraduate students, SBP, DBP, HR and state anxiety levels (a measure of anxiousness at one moment in time) were significantly higher during the reading aloud period than during the pet interaction period (see Fig. 4.17). Interaction in this study included talking to and petting the dog. While interaction with the friendly animal was less arousing than an interpersonal task the importance of touching the animal *per se* was not evaluated.

A complex experiment was designed in an attempt to clarify the role of touching an animal in moderating the stress response.[45] Sixty college students each spent 6 minutes in each of six conditions. The conditions were: resting silently with the dog absent, touching and fondling the dog without talking, calling and talking to the dog from across the room without touching it, talking to and touching the dog, having a casual conversation without the dog present and having a casual

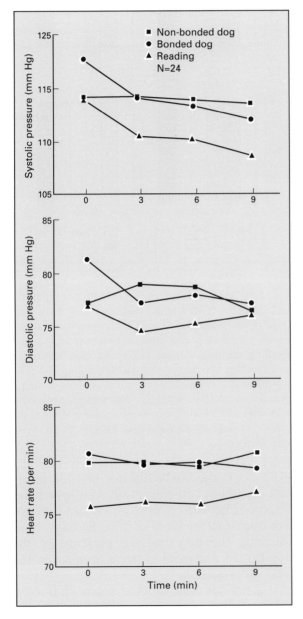

FIG. 4.16: Average systolic (top) and diastolic (middle) blood pressure and heart rate (bottom) measured at 0, 3, 6 and 9 minutes while participating in three tasks: reading quietly, petting an unfamiliar (non-bonded) dog and petting one's own dog (bonded).[5]

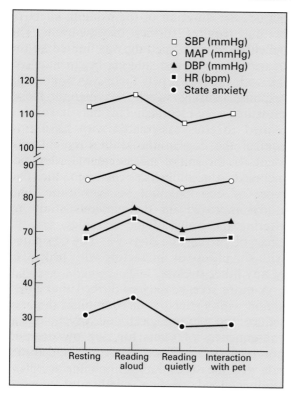

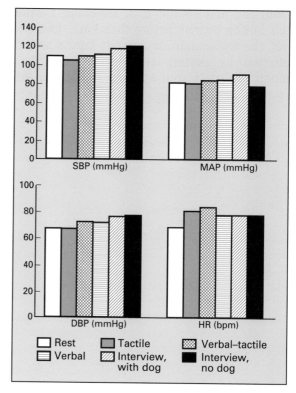

FIG. 4.17: Average mean arterial (MAP), systolic (SBP) and diastolic (DBP) blood pressures, heart rate (HR) and state anxiety during 10 minutes of the following four activities: resting quietly, reading aloud, reading quietly and petting and talking to a friendly but unfamiliar dog.[46,47]

FIG. 4.18: Average mean arterial (MAP), systolic (SBP) and diastolic (DBP) blood pressures and heart rate (HR) during 6 minutes of each of six conditions: resting silently with the dog absent (rest), touching and fondling the dog without talking (tactile), talking to and touching the dog (verbal–tactile), calling and talking to the dog from across the room (verbal), having a casual conversation with the dog present (interview, with dog) and having a casual conversation without the dog present (interview, no dog).[45]

conversation with the dog present. Blood pressure and heart rate were recorded during each of the conditions (see Fig. 4.18). To eliminate possible effects from the order of conditions, their order was assigned randomly. The results confirmed that interacting with a dog was less arousing than interacting with people. Blood pressures were significantly higher during the conversations than during the other conditions and were significantly lower while touching and fondling the dog without talking than while touching and talking to the dog and while talking to the dog without touching it. There was no difference in the cardiovascular response patterns among the 30 subjects who said they liked dogs and 30 who felt neutral about dogs. However, since none of the participants dis-

liked dogs, the study did not provide information about differences in cardiovascular responses between people who do and do not like dogs. On the basis of these findings, both touching the dog and the presence of the dog caused decreases in stress response in the laboratory setting.

It is not yet clear to what degree characteristics of the interactions, the dogs or the people determine the magnitude of the stress reducing effects. The non-judgmental aspect of interacting with a pet compared with the demands of interacting with other people is frequently cited as a possible reason for the difference in physiological responses during these interactions.[14,17,24] Speaking to an animal may be more comparable to speaking to a young child than to speaking to another adult. The characteristic slow, high pitched patterns of speech with frequent repetitions and nonsense words often used when interacting with animals or small children may be responsible for the differences in cardiovascular responses, but this possibility has not been adequately addressed.

Further research is also required to elucidate the differential effect of interacting with one's own pet and of interacting with other animals. Certainly this area of research is more difficult to standardise than the study of an animal's presence. People differ considerably in their customary interactions with their own pets. Their characteristic interactions, the strength of the relationship and the animal's behaviour in specific types of situations could all be expected to influence the physiological and psychological changes which occur during interaction. An indicator of participants' perceptions of the unfamiliar dogs might be useful in clarifying these experimental discrepancies.

Summary and Conclusions

The hypothesis that friendly animals can decrease anxiety and sympathetic nervous system arousal by providing a pleasant external focus for attention, promoting feelings of safety and providing a source of contact comfort has been supported by much of the research conducted to date. Both the presence of a friendly animal and interacting with it, have significant short term influences on physiological (i.e. blood pressure) and psychological (i.e. anxiety) indicators of stress. The presence of a friendly animal has significant impact both on pet owners and non-owners. The changes recorded have been small, but repeated throughout daily life could have a major impact on cardiovascular health. The studies showing that pet owners have reduced risk factors associated with heart disease and increased survival following release from coronary care hospitals, support this hypothesis. Since coronary heart disease and other stress related diseases are common in our society, even a small positive effect from the presence of or interaction with animals can have significant impact on the health of many individuals.

Much of the research linking pets with specific benefits has utilised dogs but there is no reason to believe that benefits are limited to specific species. In fact, the two epidemiological studies comparing pet owners and non-owners, did not find differences in the effects of pet ownership between owners of dogs and of other species.[3,15] The effectiveness of various species, breeds, or individual animals for health may well depend on personal differences in relationships with, or perceptions of animals, as well as on cultural factors.

Targeting pets to specific individuals is an area requiring additional research. In explaining the health benefits of pets for specific individuals we need to quantify the roles of relationship strength and attitudes toward animals, as well as the interrelationship between pet related variables and other sources of social support. To date, there have been no controlled studies to examine the effects of giving someone a pet on risk of developing coronary heart disease or on survival, but this type of study would be extremely difficult to carry out from both practical and ethical perspectives. It would not be possible to randomly assign individuals to take a pet. Only individuals who like pets would agree to take them and of course that would introduce bias into the sample. Furthermore, while a non-treatment control group would be possible, a placebo treatment would not. A double blind comparison, in which neither the patient nor the researcher knows who has received active and who has received inactive (placebo) treatment clearly would not be possible.

Pets should not be considered as a panacea, they will not cure cancer or hypertension. It is also important to remember that living with companion animals involves responsibilities towards that animal, in addition to any benefits that we may receive. However, benefits may be linked to these responsibilities. Owners may benefit from the establishment of structured routines for the feeding, exercising and nurturing required in animal care. Thus, we should not consider pets as drugs to be taken whenever we feel unwell but rather as having the ability to modify our lifestyle and thus enhance our health and quality of life.

References

1. Akiyama, H., Holtzman, J. M. and Britz, W. E. (1987) Pet ownership and health status during bereavement. *Omega: Journal of Death and Dying*, **17**, 187–193.
2. Allen, K. M., Blascovich, J., Tomaka, J. and Kelsey, R. M. (1991) Presence of human friends and pet dogs as moderators of autonomic responses to stress in women. *Journal of Personality and Social Psychology*, **61**, 582–589.
3. Anderson, W., Reid, P. and Jennings, G. L. (1992) Pet ownership and risk factors for cardiovascular disease. *Medical Journal of Australia*, **157**, 298–301.
4. Audy, R. J. (1971) Measurement and diagnosis of health. In *Environmental Essays on the Planet as Home*. Houghton Mifflin, Boston.
5. Baun M. M., Bergstrom, N., Langston, N. and Thoma, L. (1984) Physiological effects of human/companion animal bonding. *Nursing Research*, **50**, 126–129.
6. Beck, A. M. and Katcher, A. H. (1984) A new look at pet facilitated psychotherapy. *Journal of the American Veterinary Medical Association*, **184**, 414–421.
7. Bolin, S. E. (1987) The effects of companion animals during conjugal bereavement. *Anthrozoös*, **1**, 26–35.
8. Calhoun, D. A. (1992) Hypertension in blacks: Socioeconomic stress and sympathetic nervous system activity. *American Journal of the Medical Sciences*, **304**, 306–311.
9. Contrada, R. J. and Krantz, D. S. (1988) Stress, reactivity and Type A behavior: Current status and future directions. *Annals of Behavioral Medicine*, **10**, 64–70.
10. Fredrikson, M. (1991) Psychophysiological theories on sympathetic nervous system reactivity in the development of essential hypertension. *Scandinavian Journal of Psychology*, **32**, 254–274.
11. Friedman, M. (1969). *Pathogenesis of Coronary Artery Disease*. McGraw Hill, New York.
12. Friedmann, E. and Lockwood, R. (1991) Validation and use of the Animal Thematic Apperception Test. *Anthrozoös*, **4**, 174–183.
13. Friedmann, E. and Lockwood, R. (1993) Perception of animals and cardiovascular responses during verbalisation with an animal present. *Anthrozoös*, **6**, 115–134.
14. Friedmann, E. and Thomas, S. A. (1985) Health benefits of pets for families. Special issue: Pets and the family. *Marriage and Family Review*, **8**, 191–203.
15. Friedmann, E., Katcher, A. H., Lynch, J. J. and Thomas, S. A. (1980) Animal companions and one year survival of patients after discharge from a coronary care unit. *Public Health Reports*, **95**, 307–312.
16. Friedmann, E., Thomas, S. A., Kulick-Cuiffo, D., Lynch, J. J. and Suginohara, M. (1982) The effects of normal and rapid speech on blood pressure. *Psychosomatic Medicine*, **44**, 545–553.
17. Friedmann, E., Katcher, A. H., Thomas, S. A., Lynch, J. J. and Messent, P. R. (1983) Social interaction and blood pressure: The influence of animal companions. *Journal of Nervous and Mental Disease*, **171**, 461–465.
18. Friedmann, E., Locker, B. Z. and Thomas, S. A. (1986) Effect of the presence of a pet on cardiovascular response during communication in coronary prone individuals. Presented at Delta Society International Conference, "Living Together: People, Animals and the Environment", Boston, MA, August.
19. Garrity, T. F., Stallones, L., Marx, M. B. and Johnson, T. P. (1989) Pet ownership and attachment as supportive factors in the health of the elderly. *Anthrozoös*, **3**, 35–44.
20. Grossberg, J. M. and Alf, E. F., Jr (1985) Interaction with pet dogs: Effects on human cardiovascular response. *Journal of the Delta Society*, **2**, 20–27.
21. Grossberg, J. M., Alf, E. F., Jr and Vormbrock, J. K. (1988) Does pet dog presence reduce human cardiovascular responses to stress? *Anthrozoös*, **2**, 38–44.
22. Insel, P. M. and Roth, W. T. (1994) *Core Concepts in Health*, 7th edn. Mayfield Publishing Co., Mountainview, CA.
23. Jenkins, C. D. (1976) Recent evidence supporting psychologic and social risk factors for coronary disease. *New England Journal of Medicine*, **294**, 987–994.
24. Katcher, A. H. (1981) Interactions between people and their pets: Form and function. In *Interrelationships between People and Pets*. Ed. B. Fogle. pp. 41–67. Charles C. Thomas, Springfield, IL.
25. Katcher, A. H. and Friedmann, E. (1980) Potential health value of pet ownership. *Compendium of Continuing Education for the Veterinarian*, **2**, 117–121.

26. Katcher, A. H., Friedmann, E., Beck, A. M. and Lynch, J. J. (1983) Talking, looking and blood pressure: Physiological consequences of interaction with the living environment. In *New Perspectives on our Lives with Animal Companions*. Eds. A. H. Katcher and A. M. Beck. pp. 351–359. University of Pennsylvania Press, Philadelphia.

27. Katcher, A. H., Segal, H. and Beck, A. M. (1984) Contemplation of an aquarium for the reduction of anxiety. In *The Pet Connection: Its Influence on Our Health and Quality of Life*. Eds. R. K. Anderson, B. L. Hart and L. A. Hart. pp. 171–178. Globe Publishing Co., St Paul, MN.

28. Krantz, D. S., Helmers, K. F., Bairey, C. N., Nebel, L. E., Hedges, S. M. and Rozanski, A. (1991) Cardiovascular reactivity and mental stress-induced myocardial ischemia in patients with coronary artery disease. *Psychosomatic Medicine*, **53**, 1–12.

29. Light, K. C., Dolan, C. A., Davis, M. R. and Sherwood, A. (1992) Cardiovascular responses to an active coping challenge as predictors of blood pressure patterns 10 to 15 years later. *Psychosomatic Medicine*, **54**, 217–230.

30. Locker, B. Z. (1985) The cardiovascular response to verbalisation in Type A and Type B individuals in the presence of a dog. New York University Doctoral Dissertation, University Microfilms, Ann Arbor, MI.

31. Lockwood, R. (1983) The influence of animals on social perception. In *New Perspectives on Our Lives with Animal Companions*. Eds. A. H. Katcher and A. M. Beck. pp. 64–71. University of Pennsylvania Press, Philadelphia.

32. Lynch, J. J. (1985) *The Language of the Heart: The Human Body in Dialogue*. Basic Books, New York.

33. Mathews, K. A., Weiss, S. M., Detre, T., *et al.* (1986) *Handbook of Stress, Reactivity and Cardiovascular Disease*. Wiley, New York.

34. Messent, P. R. and Serpell, J. A. (1981) An historical and biological view of the pet–owner bond. In *Interrelationships between People and Pets*. Ed. B. Fogle. pp. 5–22. Charles C. Thomas, Springfield, IL.

35. Mugford, R. S. and M'Comisky, J. G. (1975) Therapeutic value of cage birds with old people. In *Pet Animals and Society*. Ed. R. S. Anderson. pp. 54–65. Balliere Tindall, London.

36. Ory, M. G. and Goldberg, E. L. (1983) Pet possession and life satisfaction in elderly women. In *New Perspectives on Our Lives with Animal Companions*. Eds. A. H. Katcher and A. M. Beck. pp. 303–317. University of Pennsylvania Press, Philadelphia.

37. Review panel (1981) Coronary-prone behavior and coronary heart disease: A critical review. *Circulation*, **63**, 1191–1215.

38. Robb, S. S. and Stegman, C. E. (1983) Companion animals and elderly people: A challenge for evaluators of social support. *Gerontologist*, **23**, 277–282.

39. Rosenman, R. H., Friedman, M., Straus, W., Wurm, M., Kositchek, R., Hahn, W. and Werthessen, N. T. (1964) A predictive study of coronary heart disease. *Journal of the American Medical Association*, **189**, 15–22.

40. Sebkova, J. (1977) Anxiety levels as affected by the presence of a dog. Unpublished Thesis. University of Lancaster.

41. Serpell, J. A. (1991) Beneficial effects of pet ownership on some aspects of human health. *Journal of the Royal Society of Medicine*, **84**, 717–720.

42. Siegel, J. M. (1990) Stressful life events and use of physician services among the elderly: The moderating role of pet ownership. *Journal of Personality and Social Psychology*, **58**, 1081–1086.

43. Stallones, L., Marx, M. B., Garrity, T. F. and Johnson, T. P. (1990) Pet ownership and attachment in relation to the health of U.S. adults, 21 to 64 years of age. *Anthrozoos*, **4**, 100–112.

44. Thomas, S. A. and Friedmann, E. (1990) Cardiovascular responses during verbalisation: Type A behavior and the blood pressure and heart rate responses of cardiac patients. *Nursing Research*, **39**, 48–53.

45. Vormbrock, J. K. and Grossberg, J. M. (1988) Cardiovascular effects of human–pet dog interactions. *Journal of Behavioral Medicine*, **11**, 509–517.

46. Wilson, C. C. (1987) Physiological responses of college students to a pet. *Journal of Nervous and Mental Disease*, **175**, 606–612.

47. Wilson, C. C. (1991) The pet as an anxiolytic intervention. *Journal of Nervous and Mental Disease*, **179**, 482–489.

CHAPTER 5

The Role of Pets in Therapeutic Programmes

MARY R. BURCH, LEO K. BUSTAD, SUSAN L. DUNCAN, MAUREEN FREDRICKSON and JEAN TEBAY

Historical Perspectives
LEO K. BUSTAD

People by nature are nurturers; they need nurturing as well as appropriate objects of nurture. Perhaps animals fulfil these needs. Throughout history, there appears to be an increasing dependence on nurturing and affectionate interaction. Early on, this interaction was between people and later between animals and people.[28,41] It is reasonable to speculate that wolf pups found by early man were incorporated into family life to serve as companions for some family members. This companion status was enhanced by the development of smaller canids with desirable temperament and a retention of juvenile characteristics into adulthood; referred to as **paedomorphic animals** (e.g. Cavalier King Charles Spaniels, Poodles). Early man's desire to domesticate dogs was probably influenced by the strong attachments dogs formed with people. In addition to early evidence for the use of animals as companions, there is also evidence for the historical therapeutic use of animals.

Studies of civilizations before the Judaeo-Christian era are very interesting but conclusions drawn from them must be tentative and dependent on continuing archaeological efforts. It is especially interesting to review the ancient methods of religious healing, the pagan healing gods and the significance of animals in their social structure.[27] In considering the historical role of animals in therapeutic programmes, the history of Asklepios, the Greek god of healing, is relevant. Asklepios was first mentioned by Homer (900 BC) as a 'blameless physician'. He eventually became the chief healing divinity of the Greeks. Some of his devotees were the earliest not only to develop but to record clinical observations. Asklepios' divine healing power was extended through sacred dogs (and serpents). It was believed that a person who was blind in both eyes recovered immediately after being licked by a sacred dog, since healing properties were attributed to the dog's tongue.[25] This belief is reflected in the French proverb, '*Langue de chien, sert de medicine*' (The dog's tongue serves as medicine).

For many ancient peoples there was an association between dogs and death, often with the belief that a human corpse had to be consumed by a canid in order to release the soul. Over time this belief became modified and the Zoroastrian Persian believed that a gaze from a dog could release a soul into the afterlife. Thus, amongst the Zoroastrian

Persians all dogs received respect, protection and care.[5,36]

Pliny the Elder (in the first century) and later John Keyes, a 16th-century physician, extolled the benefits of lap dogs. Keyes stated these 'delicate, neate and pretty kind of dogges called the spaniel – – gentle, or comforter,' were sought by 'dainte dames'. These dogs were often wet nursed by 'ordinary men's wives' for 'ladies of quality'.[37,38] In ancient times if a person felt in danger of going insane, he would carry a dog about with him.

In the 9th century in Gheel, Belgium, animals were introduced to benefit people who were disabled. Many Gheel residents provided extended family care to people who were disabled (a practice that still continues). Although human–animal interaction was not the main thrust of their therapeutic approach, they did implement an important animal-assisted therapy activity early in their history. In his writings of the patients of Gheel, Duval wrote, 'In this atmosphere, open in every sense, the affinities which draw man and animal together develop freely and it is on the top rank of the scale of affections, far from lacking influence on the condition of certain patients. Some interest themselves in cattle, near which they live and make their companions. There is at Gheel one patient who thinks only of birds; no one is more clever than he at catching them. Once they are caged, he leaves them no more; he leads them from his cell to the family room or when they are sunning themselves, their watchful master stands guard to protect them from the teeth of cats. Is there any doubt that these simple and childlike pleasures take away sorrows and can even help to re-establish the harmony of body and soul? Deprive this man of the company of his birds and without a doubt, his state will worsen'.[21]

Another recorded instance of introducing animals into a social therapy setting is the oft-cited York Retreat in Yorkshire, England. In the 1790s, this remarkable retreat was founded by the Society of Friends. It was the brainchild of William Tuke, a Quaker tea merchant, who was very disturbed at the treatment of patients in lunatic hospitals and asylums.[14] At the York Retreat, Tuke and his associates engaged an enlightened physician who opposed restraint and harsh drugs. Patients instead received compassionate care and concern, love, understanding and a manifestation of trust. Among the enlightened methods of treatment was the involvement of animals, including rabbits and poultry, with the thought that the patients might learn self-control by caring for the creatures dependent on them. The patients busily cared for the animals, as well as helping in the garden and learning various tasks. The York Retreat appeared to be successful and other enterprises emulated some of the practices.

Historically, the important role of pets in therapy has also been noted in nursing settings. In 1859 Florence Nightingale noted 'A small pet animal is often an excellent companion for the sick, for long chronic cases especially. A pet bird in a cage is sometimes the only pleasure of an invalid confined for years to the same room. If he can feed and clean the animal himself, he ought always to be encouraged to do so.'[35]

In 1867, 75 years after the York Retreat began operations, Bethel in Bielefeld, Germany, was founded and animals were an integral part of the enterprise. It began modestly as a home for people with epilepsy. It is now an extensive centre for the care and healing of people with disabilities. In 1977, the Bethel programme had about 5000 residents and over 5000 staff members.[9] Birds, cats, dogs and horses were evident in many of the residences and work sites from the beginning. There were also farm animals and a large wild game park. Having animals present was accepted as an appropriate and reasonable way of life. Unfortunately, there are no recorded observations of the impact of animals on Bethel patients.

The first use of animals in a USA hospital is believed to have occurred in 1919. Secretary of the Interior Franklin K. Lane wrote to Dr W. A. White, the Superintendent of St Elizabeth's Hospital in Washington, DC, suggesting that dogs be introduced for the men to 'chum and play with' and serve as a source of entertainment. Secretary Lane had been impressed with what happened to the victims of World War I. He explained his impressions as follows: 'A poor insane chap naturally reaches out for companionship and finds himself barred by the various limitations of his unfortunate associates, but he could develop a great friendship with a dog. The lonesome boys in France found their dogs a great comfort and men with shell shock recover their balance sometimes by getting close to a dog with his limited mind but his unequalled capacity for affection. Has this thing been tried in any of our institutions?'

Dr White promptly replied, stating that he'd be very glad to try it. He also stated that he knew of no systematic experimentation that had been performed, but he knew of no reason why the study should not be performed. There is no evidence to indicate that the study was ever conducted,[18] but animal visits are now routinely conducted at St Elizabeth's Hospital.

The second known use of animal-assisted therapy in hospital settings in the USA occurred in cooperation with the Red Cross in the 1940s at an Army Air Corps convalescent hospital in Pawling, New York. The Pawling Center received Air Corps personnel from every theatre of operations during World War II. The patients, convalescing from injuries or recovering from the effects of operational fatigue, were deemed to need a regime of restful activity. An academic programme was designed to keep their minds active while resting from war and its activities. As part of this experimental programme, patients were encouraged to work at the centre's farm with hogs, cattle, horses and poultry. They also benefited from the 'healing powers' of snakes, frogs, turtles. The experiment was considered successful, but it was stopped in a cost-saving move.

In the 1960s, there were some advances in developing therapeutic programmes using pets with persons with disabilities. In 1966, a rehabilitation centre for people with disabilities was established in central Norway. It was named Beitostolen; the motivating forces for its establishment were Erling Stordahl (who was blind) and his wife, Anna, who believed

a new approach for providing therapy was needed for people who were disabled. Along with a physiotherapy and sports programme, the centre also had dogs and horses as an important component of the therapy regimen. People who were blind learned to ski and ride horses. This very impressive and successful programme continues today.[14]

After World War II, some efforts were directed at involving companion animals in clinical psychology therapy settings. Dr Boris Levinson, a clinical psychologist at Yeshiva University, accidentally discovered that a companion animal could be helpful in therapy for a disturbed child. The accidental meeting of Levinson's dog and a child who was referred to him for treatment, was the key to eventual rehabilitation of the patient. On the basis of this success, Dr Levinson promoted the interaction of carefully selected companion animals for facilitating therapy. His plea for rigorous research to establish boundaries and principles was accompanied by caution regarding how to select and train animals for this work.[10,11,14,29,30] Sam and Elizabeth Corson and their associates took up Levinson's charge, in their work at Ohio State University. They attempted systematically to evaluate animal-assisted therapy and realised substantial success.[16,17]

No matter what the setting, one of the recurring admirable traits discussed throughout history is the fidelity of dogs. When one considers the remarkable role that animals have played in therapeutic settings in the last century, the words that Lorenz wrote pertaining to dogs are especially meaningful: 'The fidelity of a dog is a precious gift demanding no less binding moral responsibility than the friendship of a human being. The bond with a true dog is as lasting as the ties of this Earth can ever be, a fact which should be noted by anyone who decides to acquire a canine friend.'[31]

Animal-Assisted Therapy
MARY R. BURCH

Beginning in the 1980s, professionals who used animals in therapeutic settings began to make a distinction between animal-assisted activities (AAA) and animal-assisted therapy (AAT). As the level of professionalism increased for these therapists, previously used terms such as 'pet therapy' and 'pet-facilitated therapy' began to be abandoned in favour of terms that did not suggest that simply any pet could perform therapy work. As the field continues to advance, there is an increasing awareness with regard to selecting animals for use in therapy that have met specific screening and training criteria.

AAA provide opportunities for motivational, educational, recreational, and/or therapeutic benefits to enhance quality of life and are delivered in a variety of therapeutic environments by a specially trained professional or volunteer, in association with animals.[19]

AAT is a goal-directed intervention in which an animal is used as an integral part of the treatment process. The therapy is directed or delivered by a health service professional with specialised expertise.[19] While the results of AAA may often be characterised by happy times and good feelings, the results of AAT are both observable and measurable. The goals of an AAT programme may be to increase desirable behaviours, or to decrease inappropriate behaviours. In the AAT context, animals are now used in many therapeutic settings, including prisons, nursing homes, developmental disabilities facilities, settings for people with physical handicaps, programmes for people with head injuries, hospices, AIDS programmes, schools and individualised therapy sessions. Therapists have used animals for a variety of purposes from treating clinical problems such as phobias, teaching new skills such as walking and talking and increasing appropriate social behaviours.

Increasing Appropriate Social Behaviours

A successful prison-based AAT programme was started in 1975 by David Lee in Lima, Ohio (USA). In a research programme that involved cats, goats, birds and small farm animals, Lee demonstrated that inmates who had pets to care for were less violent, had increased appropriate social behaviours, fewer infractions and needed less medication than those inmates without pets.[7]

Similar positive results were seen when dogs were used at the Purdy Treatment Center, a Washington maximum security prison for women. In the Purdy programme, dogs were placed with inmates who had been selected as dog trainers. Some of the Purdy dogs were placed in homes as pets, but others received advanced training by the inmates and were placed as assistance animals for people with disabilities. The Purdy programme met the definition of AAT by teaching functional vocational skills such as grooming, dog care, veterinary assistance and kennel management. Purdy inmates who were interviewed about the programme often reported increases in self-esteem and the ability to feel better about themselves as a result of being able to make a contribution by training an animal for service work.[33]

Teaching New Skills and Reducing Maladaptive Behaviours

Animals can be used in therapy settings to teach new skills or to reduce maladaptive behaviours. The following case study demonstrates how animals were used as contingent reinforcers to decrease tantrums and to teach a child to walk.

Kevin was a 3-year-old boy who was prenatally exposed to drugs including cocaine and heroin. He was referred for behavioural assistance because of excessive tantrums and resisting the touch of other people to the extent that his mother had difficulty giving him a bath. He could stand but would not attempt to walk and his physiotherapist felt that this was due to a lack of motivation. An assessment of potential behavioural reinforcers was conducted but Kevin did not respond to any of the traditional reinforcers for young children such as toys, music, or food. One day, thinking that Kevin might respond in a new setting, he was taken to the beach. He began to point and make noises when he saw a seagull, the first signs of any expressive communication. A cockatiel was introduced into the home setting as a contingent reinforcer for appropriate bath time behaviour. Immediately following each short bathing session where there was no tantrum, Kevin was rewarded with a visit to the cockatiel. In a matter of weeks, Kevin was allowing his mother to bathe him with no tantrums and in the seventh session, he said his first word, 'bird'.[6]

The dramatic response to the bird led to the assessment of Kevin's reaction to a trained, certified, therapy dog. Kevin was very interested in the dog and he initiated contact by reaching out to stroke it. Once the dog was established as a reinforcer, a 10 stage programme was developed to teach walking. The stages ranged from crawling to the dog, to walking to the dog without assistance. In the first 10 therapy sessions, Kevin acquired the first four stages of the programme. In the eleventh therapy session, Kevin took his first two steps towards the dog and by the end of the session, had walked nearly 2 metres in order to greet the dog. This case demonstrates how animals can be used in therapy settings to both teach new skills (e.g. walking) and to reduce or eliminate maladaptive behaviours (e.g. tantrums during self-care routines).[6]

Using Animals in Clinical Settings

Animals have also been used effectively in clinical psychology settings. In a study conducted in conjunction with the Bayley Seton Hospital in New York, certified therapy dogs were used to work with two autistic teenagers who were dog-phobic. The phobic response reduced the quality of life for these teenagers as it became difficult for them to be taken for walks in the community. A programme of exposure to increasingly strong stimuli was developed, with 13 stages ranging from entering the room with a dog 6 metres away to holding the end of a leash and stroking the dog. The dog used was a trained therapy animal. Sessions progressed until the teenagers were

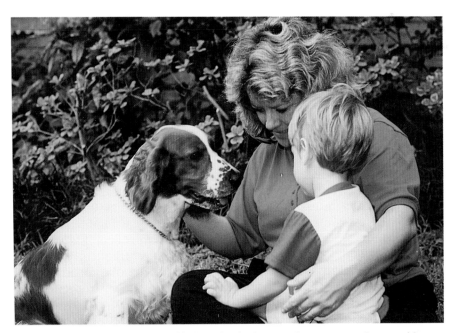

FIG. 5.1: The use of certified, trained, therapy dogs can produce rapid results in therapeutic settings.

comfortable with stroking the first therapy dog, then a second dog was introduced and eventually the students were taken for walks to see dogs in the neighbourhood.[8] Prior to this work many studies showed effective results with the standard procedures used to treat phobias (e.g. systematic desensitization, modelling and reinforcement). The unique aspect of this treatment of dog phobia was the use of trained, certified, therapy dogs. This meant that the dogs could be relied upon to stay in one place without moving, if instructed to do so. It was therefore possible for the handlers to prevent the animals from making unpredictable movements, which would scare the participants and reduce treatment progress.

New Applications of AAT

As the field of AAT continues to develop, the applications are expanding. In recent years, animal-assisted therapy has been used effectively with children who have had prenatal exposure to drugs, as a result of their mothers using substances such as crack, cocaine, or heroin during pregnancy. These children often have health, neurological and behavioural problems, attention deficits and language or other developmental delays. Often socially withdrawn and resistive to touch, many of these children will respond to an animal in an AAT setting,[6] as the following case study demonstrates.

A four-year-old child who was clinically hyperactive, substance-exposed, blind and mentally retarded was referred for treatment. She concentrated on tasks for less than a minute at a time and at home engaged in destructive behaviour. Her mother reported that she could not leave her unsupervised for even a few seconds. An assessment of potential reinforcers was conducted and it was discovered that the child would become quiet when she was stroking a therapy dog. A programme was developed where the child was given the chance to stroke the dog while a children's music show was on television. Eventually, the dog was replaced with a stuffed animal and the child would play with the toy and listen to music for 30 minutes at a time.[22]

A larger scale AAT project involving children with hyperactivity was implemented at the Philadelphia Devereux Foundation. Fifty boys aged 9–15 were selected as participants for the study, based on their consistent failure in school, behaviour problems and psychiatric conditions. The participants were randomly split into two groups. One group was assigned to non-animal activities such as rock climbing. The second group was assigned to the Companionable Animal Zoo, where they learned about and cared for a variety of animals for 5 hours per week. The author of the study reported that, 'Exposure to the animals seemed not only to reduce symptoms of hyperactivity and what we call 'conduct disorder,' but it also increased the children's learning capabilities'.[24]

As the applications of AAT continue to expand, the field is witnessing an increase in professionalism. There are training and certification programmes for volunteers, instructors and animals and some colleges are offering AAT course work. Once primarily a volunteer activity, the therapeutic potential of AAT is becoming recognised and AAT services are now purchased in some therapy settings. As we approach the next century, there is a growing recognition that in many cases, animal-assisted therapy is the treatment of choice.

Animal-Assisted Activities
MAUREEN FREDRICKSON

People living in institutional settings such as nursing homes, hospitals, rehabilitation centres, residential educational programmes and correctional facilities have all aspects of daily life controlled. Individuals who live in such facilities frequently experience depression, anxiety, isolation and other symptoms associated with institutionalisation.[20] When animals and their care become a part of the routine in a treatment facility, it has been noted that both staff and residents can benefit. An opportunity to nurture animals

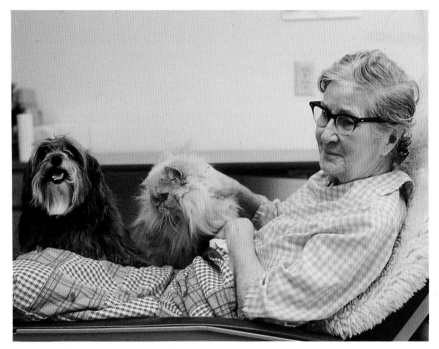

FIG. 5.2: Animals can reduce feelings of isolation and loneliness in
therapeutic settings.

often mitigates the artificial quality of institutional settings. Animals provide an opportunity for play, intimacy, nurturing and socialisation.

Programmes providing contact with companion animals can include components of an individual's treatment or a wider approach where animals are present in institutional settings to enhance the quality of life for both residents and staff. The most common method for incorporating animals into the lives of people living in institutional settings is through animal-assisted activity programmes. In an informal and non-data-based manner, AAA frequently incorporate goals that affect quality of life issues for individuals served by the programme. Goals may include: reduced feelings of isolation, decreased depression, reduced anxiety and increased socialisation.

AAA are defined as programmes that 'provide opportunities for motivational, educational, or recreational benefits to enhance the quality of life'.[19] Such programmes are delivered in a variety of settings, require minimal documentation and less staff involvement than animal-assisted therapy programmes. Animals chosen for AAA must meet specific criteria including: being in good health, free of external and internal parasites, and demonstrating appropriate skills and temperament for interacting with the special needs of specific populations. The programmes are divided into passive or interactive programmes and include both visiting and residential animals.

Passive Animal-Assisted Activities

Perhaps the most easily recognised forms of AAA introduce an aquarium or small caged birds (such as finches or canaries) into medical or dental waiting rooms. The bright colour of the fish and the soothing sound of bubbling water, or the sounds and activities of birds can direct a patient's attention away from their appointment. Aquaria and caged birds also provide staff with relief from workplace pressures, as they take time out to watch or care for the animals.

The role of animals in these settings is passive as people do not handle the animals, but there can be positive effects from simply having an animal present. In rehabilitation units for geriatric adults, the presence of companion birds has been shown to decrease significantly the depression of older residents.[2] Another benefit of the passive nature of these programmes is that the animals require minimal screening. Ensuring that animals are disease-free and free of parasites is usually sufficient.

Other cost-effective AAA that provide excellent motivational and recreational benefits are those that create outdoor bird feeding stations and gardens that attract butterflies and other animals. Some facilities set up microphones on outdoor feeders to give non-ambulatory residents the opportunity to listen to bird song. A room for observing the birds provides residents with a place to socialise with other residents, as well as with family members. The use of this type of programme is increasing and is particularly helpful in hospice or Alzheimer care programmes, where family members may need help in focusing conver-sations. In 1992, approximately 70% of the hospices in the UK and Ireland who responded to a survey reported having resident pets.[4]

Interactive Animal-Assisted Activities

More interactive types of AAA include residential companion animal programmes or visiting pet programmes. In residential programmes, the animals live at the facility with care provided by staff or residents. Visiting pet programmes allow specially screened and trained owners and their animals to enter the facility at a specific time and date, for a fixed period of time. Visiting animals may include rabbits, cats, dogs, pigs and llamas. Although these programmes are more restrictive than residential animal programmes, animal visits are more appropriate in facilities where staff members are involved with in-depth resident care (such as in hospices or hospitals), in facilities where proper care of resident animals would be insufficient, or where there is a high turnover of staff or residents. Volunteer training and animal screening is critical to

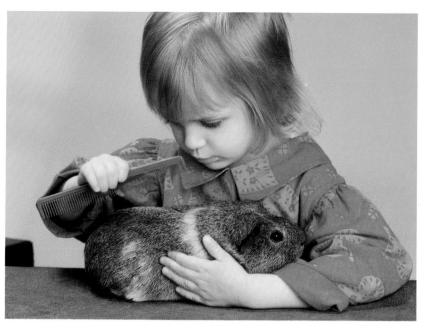

FIG. 5.3: Small animals such as guinea pigs provide diversion from routine care and they can facilitate nurturing activities.

the success of AAA. Volunteers must understand their role in helping their animal safely negotiate health care equipment such as wheelchairs and intravenous tubes, as well as feeling comfortable sharing their pet with people who are ill or disabled.

Programmes that involve individuals in pet care often motivate people to interact with others, increase physical activity and provide an opportunity to learn life skills. The animals provide residents with some diversion from routine care and allow them to engage in nurturing activities. In the UK, caring for birds has been shown to have a therapeutic effect on inmates serving prison sentences. Relationships between staff and inmates improved as a result of working together to care for the birds and inmates who were involved in bird care show less abuse toward others.[34]

Residential AAA require consideration of the animal's needs: its ability to cope in an institutional setting, its needs for safety, housing, food and rest. Dogs are therefore not an ideal choice for these programmes because they require training, regular exercise and rely on one person for leadership. Many dog mascot programmes have been discontinued due to animal behaviour problems, obesity, attachment to one person, or a lack of an ongoing specific person to care for the dog.[20] Cats, rabbits and other small mammals have been more successful when used in indoor residential programmes.

Educational opportunities provided through AAA include programmes in schools, juvenile detention facilities, residential educational programmes and correctional facilities. A significant number of correctional facilities in the USA and Europe have developed programmes in which inmates care for small pets, fish and livestock as part of vocational training.[12] A number of programmes work co-operatively with local animal shelters to train dogs for placement as companions for seniors or as service dogs for people with disabilities. Programmes also provide residents and staff with opportunities to step out of the facility routine and see each other in positive ways. AAA can provide family members with a focus for visits and provide unlimited positive opportunities for volunteer involvement. The long term benefit of AAA is very often a reduction in the stress and depression encountered in institutional programmes that do not use animals as a part of the therapeutic process.

Service Dogs
SUSAN L. DUNCAN

Dogs have been serving humans for thousands of years. They have assisted in gathering food by chasing, flushing and retrieving quarry, protected livestock, and provided warmth and companionship. As our societies and environments have changed, we have continued to evaluate the dogs' talents and find new ways to incorporate them into our lifestyles.

Recent medical advancements have made it possible for people to live longer in spite of

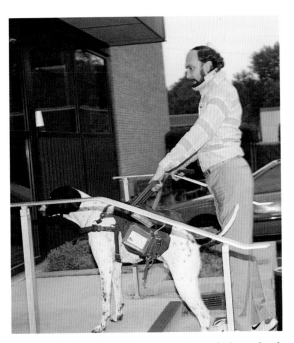

FIG. 5.4: Service dogs help owners live as independently as possible by assisting in balance, carrying items and helping throughout the day with physical tasks. Courtesy of the Delta Society

conditions which substantially limit activity. People with disabilities are now encouraged to become as functional as possible and society has responded, albeit slowly, in the accommodation of individuals with disabilities. Thus, this century has generated yet another role for canines: that of **service dog**.

The term 'service dogs' does not indicate any military connections, nor are the animals merely pets who enjoy extended travel privileges. Service dogs are dogs which are specifically trained to help individuals overcome the limitations of their disabilities. These dogs can and do replace human helpers and can be trained reliably to perform a number of tasks that are specific to their owner's needs.

The concept of service dogs is not new. No one knows when the first service dog was trained, but organised efforts to provide dogs capable of guiding blind people began in Germany during World War I.[40] Eventually, dogs were found to be equally helpful to people with other types of disabilities. **Hearing dogs**, **seizure-alert dogs** and **assistance dogs** have joined the professional ranks of the **guide dogs** and in 1990 the term service dog was coined in the USA to describe any dog individually trained to do work or perform tasks for the benefit of a person with a disability.[42] The use of this single term is beneficial for two reasons: first, it simplifies the identification process for these working dogs and, second, it helps avoid undesired disclosure of a person's medical condition during that identification process. For example, a person entering a place where dogs are usually not permitted (such as a restaurant) need only state that the dog is a service dog. At the present time, in the USA the dog is not required to wear an identification badge and the person is not required to discuss the type of work the dog does. Thus, the person's privacy is protected and a measure of dignity and decorum can be maintained. Other countries differ with respect to the rules concerning access of service dogs, but in many areas the traditional 'Guide Dog Only' signs are being replaced by those indicating access for all service dogs.

Service dogs may be any breed, size or colour and in some cases may not wear any identifying equipment, such as a harness, backpack, or special collar or leash. The important issues pertaining to these animals is that they are able reliably to perform the tasks necessary to meet the human's needs without being disruptive or destructive. Dogs can be trained reliably to perform many tasks. These include the traditional roles of leading people who have visual impairments so they can safely navigate their environments, alerting people who have hearing impairments to the presence of people and specific sounds, and the more recent activities of helping physically by picking up things (retrieving), providing balance or support for walking, carrying items in backpacks and opening doors. The most recent type of service involves sensing their owners' oncoming seizures and warning them. The person with epilepsy (seizure disorder) then has time to sit or lie down before the seizure begins. This task been developed since the discovery that some dogs are able to detect an oncoming seizure in a person before that person was aware of it. The dogs initially may only make small responses to the impending seizure, but can be trained to give recognisable signals. Some dogs can even distinguish between the different forms of seizure that their owner may have. The method by which the dogs detect seizures is not understood at present and requires further research.

It has been suggested that service dogs may provide benefit to their owners in addition to their physical aid but this has not been quantified or qualified to a great extent. Research has shown many benefits of bonded pet ownership, such as lowered blood pressure and heart rate. The stewardship issue alone (which involves providing for the care and daily maintenance needs of the dog) can provide responsibility that helps a person achieve more positive interactions with his or her environment. Anecdotal reports of the effects of service dogs by their owners and significant others have included physical, psychological and social benefits. The benefits received are likely to vary depending on the physical condition of the owner. Reports have suggested that in addition to the physical aid, owners can receive enhanced confidence and self-esteem, an increased sense of trust and personal security and a decreased sense of loneliness and frustration. The dogs also reduce a person's dependency on other humans and assistance devices and reduced worry on the part of significant others regarding the owner's moment-to-moment well-being. A further benefit may be the ability of an animal to divert attention from the disability and provide a non-disease oriented focus for the owners and others.

The following case studies also illustrate the scope of the service dog's value.

Ms D had multiple sclerosis. She was 38 years old, married, with two children. Her continual symptoms included left-sided muscle weakness, mild to moderate coordination problems, ataxia and poor balance, numbness and fatigue. Prior to obtaining a service dog, Ms D had limited her activity to reduce the possibility of injuries from accidents and had curtailed her participation in many activities (involvement at children's schools, performing simple errands, showering when no one else was home, etc.). However after acquiring a service dog, there were some positive changes in Ms D's ability to live more independently. The service dog assisted Ms D by helping her up and down steps and ramps, providing balance and momentum. It reduced the amount of bending over and lifting that Ms D had to perform by bringing the telephone or other designated items to her; it guided her safely in and out of the home when her vision was impaired and provided a sense of protection if she had to rest in a public area. In addition to a greater level of self confidence, Ms D reported a 75% reduction in the amount of time that she spent in her motorised wheelchair, due to the service dog's ability to help her walk.

In another case, Mr B was a 13-year-old boy with cerebral palsy. He lived with his parents and attended a public junior high school. He had difficulty with balance, mobility, coordination and speech. A service dog was acquired to help him with walking, carrying items, rising from falls, opening doors and some retrieval. Following acquisition, Mr B's mother reported a significant increase in his socialisation. The increase in socialisation was attributed to several factors which included: the attraction of the dog as a point of interest with his peers, a reduction in the time that a parent or care-giver was in attendance, and an increase in Mr B's self-confidence. A noted improvement in his speech also occurred as he learnt to communicate verbally with his service dog. A reduction in Mr B's spasticity and improvement in his muscle strength and co-ordination were attributed to his increased mobility and the physical care of his service dog.

A third case in which a service dog made a dramatic difference in a person's quality of life, concerns Ms L, a single 37-year-old who had seizure disorders. Prior to utilising her service dog, Ms L experienced many accidents secondary to her uncontrolled seizures; for example, she was struck by a car when a seizure occurred while she was crossing a road and she walked through a plate glass window and severed an artery during another seizure. The service dog was trained to predict the uncontrolled seizures and alert Ms L prior to their occurrence. She was then able to assume a safe position for the duration of the seizures. The service dog stayed with Ms L during the seizure, providing protection during the unconscious period. As a result of obtaining the service dog, Ms L can now travel about freely without fear of physical harm or humiliation due to the effects of her seizures.

In one of the few studies of the benefits of service animals, disabled children visited a busy shopping area both with and without their service dogs. When the dogs were present, the children received more friendly contact from passers-by than did the same children without their dogs.[32]

A more recent study has shown that the presence of a service dog results in improvements in the user's psychological well-being, self-esteem and community integration.[1] Further, service dog users have reported requiring an average of 72% fewer hours of personal assistant time.[1] In addition to giving individuals a greater sense of independence, reductions in the amount of time a personal assistant is required reduces the cost of care, which can more than offset the cost of the dog's training and care. In some cases the financial savings amounted to several hundred US dollars per week.[1]

Any person with a disability which significantly affects one or more major life function may benefit from a service dog. If the quality of a persons' life can be improved by the delegation of tasks to a service dog, that person is a prime candidate for service dog referral. However, the decision to obtain an animal involves making a lifestyle commitment and must be the potential owner's choice. Methods for obtaining a service dog include getting a dog already trained by an established programme, getting a dog that is trained by an individual, or self-training a dog with or without assistance. However, it is crucial that the service dog is trained to supply assistance relative to the person's individual needs and that the person is capable of integrating the

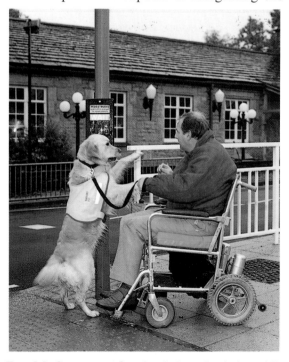

FIG. 5.5: Owners can function independently in public settings with the assistance of service dogs. Reproduced with permission from © The Picture Box on behalf of Support Dogs.

service dog into their lifestyle.

In the USA, Federal (i.e. *Americans with Disabilities Act, 1990*) and State laws permit people with disabilities to be accompanied by their service dogs in places of public accommodation.[42] Service dogs work not only in the home but can provide assistance to their owners on a 24 hour basis. Service dogs can be found working with their owners in a wide variety of settings, from restaurants and retail stores, to hospitals and dental clinics. At the present time, service dog programmes are perhaps most diverse and advanced in the USA, but other countries have recognised the importance of developing quality service dog programmes and advances are being made in many areas. Currently, demand for service animals is usually greater than their availability, but hopefully this position will change in the next few years.

Therapeutic Riding
MARY R. BURCH AND JEAN TEBAY

Therapeutic horseback riding plays an important part in the history of using animals in therapeutic programmes. Horseback riding for people with disabilities has been mentioned in the literature for centuries. The Greeks, perhaps as early as 500 BC, gave horseback rides to individuals who were considered untreatable or incurable, in order to improve their spirits[8] and by the 18th and 19th centuries, the medical literature described the therapeutic benefits of riding.

One of the first studies noting the benefits of riding horses was performed by Chassigne in Paris in 1870. He observed that riding was most beneficial in the treatment of hemiplegia, paraplegia and other neurological disorders. He specifically noted an improvement in posture, balance, joint movement and muscle control that he ascribed to the active and passive movements provided by the horse. Recent observations confirm these benefits.[10,13,15] A survey conducted in 1982 showed that the UK, West Germany and the USA had all been using horses specifically to benefit people with disabilities for about 20 years.[39] Today, world-wide, approximately 30 countries practice some form of therapeutic riding. International congresses sponsored by the Federation for Riding for the Disabled are held every three years and training and standards now exist for professionals in this field.

Therapeutic riding is the term used to describe all of the various uses of the horse to improve the quality of life for people with disabilities. There are many forms of therapeutic riding but they generally fall into three separate categories. The first is riding as an adapted sport or recreation. Here, riding instructors with additional specialised training in the therapeutic uses of the horse, teach riding as a skill to individuals with a variety of disabilities. The benefits of this adapted sport are not only the pleasure and fun of participating in recreational activity, but also

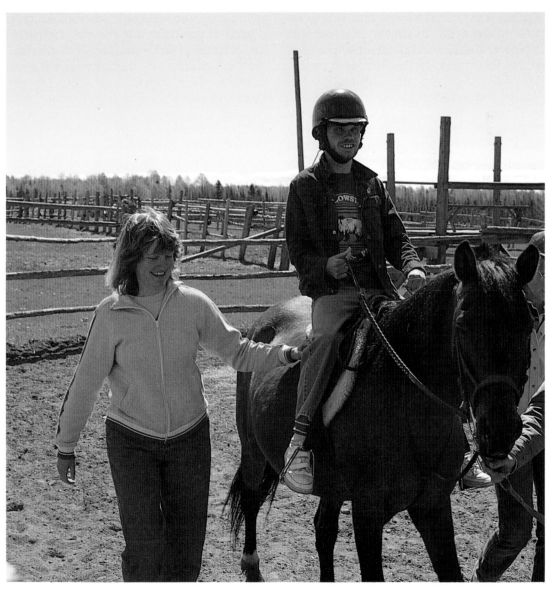

FIG. 5.6: Therapeutic riding can result in improvements in posture, balance, mobility and overall functioning. Courtesy of the Delta Society.

include psychological components. Riding gives the disabled person a new perspective and an increased feeling of self-esteem and well-being. Driving horses is also recognised as an adapted sport for people with disabilities. Many clients who are unable to mount or sit on the horse find that they are able to drive specially constructed vehicles pulled by the horse. This sport is growing rapidly as an alternative to riding.

In the second category, remedial riding, professionals (e.g. psychologists, special education teachers) use the horse and riding setting to enhance the treatment environment. This type of riding is conducted using a team approach incorporating the treatment professional and the specially trained riding instructor and is probably the most common type of therapeutic riding. The emphasis in these programmes is to teach not only functional riding skills, but also to incorporate therapeutic goals into the programme. The programme may address goals that are educational, behavioural, psychological, or physical in nature.[39] For example, in addition to skills learned related to riding horses, in a study involving children with cerebral palsy, a specific treatment goal was to improve balance.[3] In Germany, gymnastic sports vaulting (gymnastic manoeuvres performed on horseback) is used with emotionally disturbed adolescents. The main objective is to correct the child's behaviour problems and to facilitate interactions with peers. Up to six children may participate in a group with one vaulting horse and the child's ability to function within the group is stressed as well as achievement, physical co-ordination, self-confidence and courage.

The final category is the use of the horse in medical settings to treat patients with physical dysfunction. This use of the horse is called **hippotherapy**, which literally means 'treatment with the help of the horse' (from the Greek word for horse, *eohippos*). The professional who directs or delivers this therapy complies with professional legal and ethical requirements. Incorporating horses as a treatment option requires that the professional has specialised expertise about horses.

In this setting, the therapist (who is an occupational or physiotherapist) positions the patient on the horse during treatment, analyses the responses to the moving horse and directs the movement of the horse. The goal of hippotherapy is to improve the patient's posture, balance, mobility and function.[39]

While the field of therapeutic riding has advanced significantly in the last few decades, there is a lack of empirical research to validate the effects of riding as a treatment modality. The literature on horse selection, techniques for therapy sessions and case reports is growing, but there is a great need for studies which analyse the efficacy of specific aspects of therapeutic riding and compare their effects with other forms of treatment.

Acknowledgements—The editorial support and source selection of Charlene Douglas, Daun Martin, Pam Barker, Signe Bustad and Lacy Carson for the Historical Perspectives portion of this chapter is gratefully acknowledged.

References

1. Allen, K. (1994) Physical disability and assistance dogs: quality of life issues. Proceedings of the Delta Society 13th Annual Conference, New York.
2. Baun, M., Cardiello, F. and Jassen, J. (1992) The use of avian companionship to alleviate the depression, loneliness and low morale during translocation of the older adult into a skilled rehabilitation unit. Proceedings of the 6th International Conference: Animals and Us, Montreal, Canada.
3. Bertoti, D. B. (1988) Effect of therapeutic horseback riding on posture in children with cerebral palsy. *Physical Therapy*, **68**, 1505–1512.
4. Biswas, B. and Ahmedzai, S. (1992) Companion animals in British hospices. Proceedings of the 6th International Conference: Animals and Us, Montreal, Canada.
5. Boyd, J. and Rollin, B. (1994) Personal communication.
6. Burch, M. R. (1991) Animal-assisted therapy and crack babies: A new frontier. *Pet Partners Newsletter*.
7. Burch, M. R. (1994) The world's best therapists have wet noses. *Bloodlines*, **76**, 52–54.

8. Burch, M. R., Lettis, A. and Gill, M. J. (1991) *Conquering Dog Phobia: Dogs, Data and Dogma.* Behavior Management Consultants, Inc., Tallahassee, FL.

9. Bustad, L. K. (1978) The peripatetic dean: Bethel visit. *Western Veterinarian*, **16 (3)**, 2.

10. Bustad, L. K. (1980a) *Animals, Aging and the Aged.* University of Minnesota Press. Minneapolis.

11. Bustad, L. K. (1980b) The veterinarian and animal-facilitated therapy. Proceedings of the 47th Annual Meeting of the American Animal Hospital Association (John V. Lacroix Lecture).

12. Bustad, L. K. (1990) *Compassion: Our Last Great Hope.* Delta Society, Renton, Washington.

13. Bustad, L. K. (1993) Health benefits of human–animal interaction. In *Aging in Good Health.* Eds. F. Lieberman and M. F. Collen. Plenum Press, New York.

14. Bustad, L. K. and Hines, L. M. (1984) Historical perspectives of the human–animal bond. In *The Pet Connection.* Eds. R. K. Anderson, B. L. Hart and L. A. Hart.

15. Chassigne, R. (1870) Physiologie de l'equitation de son application a l'hygiene et a la therapeutique. MD dissertation: Paris. (National Library Science microfilm No. 75–88).

16. Corson, S. A., Corson, E., Corson, O. L. and Gwynne, P. H. (1975) Pet facilitated psychotherapy. In *Pet Animals and Society.* Ed. R. S. Anderson. Williams and Wilkins, Baltimore.

17. Corson, S. A., Corson, E., Corson, O. L., Gwynne, P. H. and Arnold, L. E. (1977) Pet dogs as non-verbal communication links in hospital psychiatry. *Comprehensive Psychiatry*, **18**, 61–72.

18. D'Amore, A. R. T. and Eckburg, A. L. (1976) William Alanson White: The Washington years: 1903–1937. Washington, DC: USA Department of Health Education and Welfare, Public Health Service, National Institute of Mental Health, St Elizabeth's Hospital.

19. Delta Society (1992) Pet partners: Helping animals help people with animal-assisted activities workshop manual. Delta Society, Renton, WA.

20. Delta Society (1992–94) Informal review of nursing homes in the USA that obtained a dog for a mascot. 1992–94. Delta Society, Renton, Washington.

21. Duval, M. J. (1860) Gheel, ou une colonie d'alienes vivant en famille et en liberté: étude sur le meileur mode d'assistance et de traitement dans les maladies mentales. Paris: Guillaumin, et. cie.

22. Fraser, J. (1991) A lesson in healing. *American Kennel Gazette*, New York.

23. Glasow, B. and Spink, J. (1982) Therapeutic riding in the United States. Paper presented at the Fourth International Congress on Therapeutic Riding, Hamburg, West Germany.

24. Golin, M. and Walsh, T. (1994) Heal emotions with fur, feathers and love. *Prevention Magazine*, December.

25. Halliday, W. R. (1922) Animal pets in Greece. *Discovery*, **3**, 151–154.

26. Heipertz, W. (1977) *Therapeutic Riding, Medicine, Education and Sports.* Greenbelt Riding Association, Ottawa, Canada.

27. Jayne, W. A. (1962) *The Healing Gods of Ancient Civilizations.* pp. 193–195. University Books, Inc., New York.

28. Katcher, A. H. and Beck, A. M. (1991) Animal companions. In *Man and Beast Revisted.* Eds. M. H. Robinson and L. Tiger. Smithsonian Institution Press, Washington, DC.

29. Levinson, B. M. (1969) *Pet-Oriented Child Psychotherapy.* Charles Thomas, Springfield, IL.

30. Levinson, B. M. (1972) *Pets and Human Development.* Charles C. Thomas, Springfield, IL.

31. Lorenz, K. Z. (1953) *Man meets Dog.* Penguin Books, New York.

32. Mader, B., Hart, L. A. and Bergin, B. (1989) Social acknowledgements for children with disabilities: Effects of service dogs. *Child Development*, **60**, 1529–1534.

33. Maggitti, P. (1988) Nor iron bars a cage: The story of pets in prison. *The Animal's Agenda*, July/August, 26–29.

34. Mead, A. (1992) Prisons — therapeutic benefits of birds. Proceedings of the 6th International Conference: Animals and Us, Montreal, Canada.

35. Nightingale, F. (1859) (reprinted in 1946). *Notes on Nursing: What it is and What it is not.* Harrison and Sons, London.

36. Schwabe, C. W. (1994) Animals in the Ancient World. In *Animals and Human Society: Changing Perspectives.* Eds. A. Manning and J. Serpell. Routledge, London.

37. Serpell, J. A. (1986) *In the Company of Animals.* Basil Blackwell, New York.

38. Smithcors, J. F. (1960) Veterinariana: Lap of luxury. *Modern Veterinary Practice*, **41(6)**, 68.

39. Spink, J. (1993) *Developmental Riding Therapy: A Team Approach to Assessment and Treatment. Therapy Skills Builders.* Tuscan, Arizona.

40. Stuckey, K. (1982) Guide dog. *The World Book Encyclopedia*, **8G**, 408.

41. Tanner, N. M. (1988) *On Becoming Human.* Cambridge University Press, New York.

42. United States Department of Justice (1990) The Americans with Disabilities Act. Title III, Article 4: Washington, DC.

CHAPTER 6

Avoiding Problems: The Importance of Socialisation

SANDRA McCUNE, JUSTINE A. McPHERSON and JOHN W. S. BRADSHAW

Introduction

A well adjusted and sociable pet reciprocates the affection it receives from its owner. The key to ensuring such a rewarding companion is adequate socialisation, particularly during the crucial first weeks of life. Socialisation is the process by which an animal develops appropriate social behaviour. Cats and dogs differ from most mammalian species in that they can be simultaneously socialised to their own species and to people. If effort is committed at this early stage, the benefits are tremendous in terms of the quality of the pet–owner relationship as it develops. Breeders, both professional and casual, have a responsibility to give the animals they produce the best chance of developing into rewarding pets. This chapter focuses on the importance of socialisation for the development of normal, well adjusted behaviour in cats and dogs.

An extraordinary degree of trust and intimacy can be observed between people and their pets. The willingness of cats and dogs to submit themselves to the whims of their owners differs enormously among individuals but largely depends on their early socialisation, temperament and early environment.[41] Adequate socialisation of the kitten or puppy has enormous value in preventing the development, later in life, of inappropriate behaviour and deficits of character that can seriously detract from the pleasures of pet ownership. The break-down of the relationship can literally be life threatening for the pet as behavioural problems are one of the most common reasons cited for euthanasia.[14]

Socialisation improves the trainability of dogs in at least two distinct ways. Familiarity with people promotes learning of interactive tasks, such as walking on a leash and staying in the 'down' position. In addition, a varied environment, which is normally a natural concomitant of the socialisation process, is responsible for producing puppies which have superior problem-solving abilities.[58] Likewise, kittens raised in a stimulating environment perform better in discrimination tasks[44] and are less likely to show fearful and disorganised behaviour than are kittens raised in individual cages.[59]

The result of inadequate socialisation is an animal which cannot relax and enjoy life,

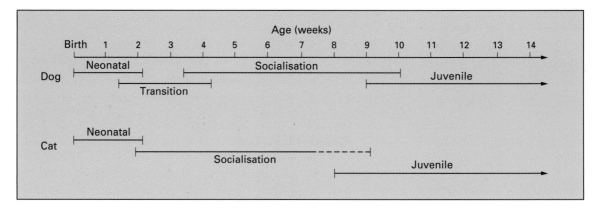

FIG. 6.1: Duration of the phases of development in the dog and cat.

that is susceptible to stress and which may be threatened by even such simple events as having visitors to the house. Inadequately socialised kittens and puppies are often intolerant of close contact with people or other animals and may even threaten them. The typical noisy, unpredictable movements of children may be perceived as particularly threatening and make the unsocialised pet a danger to them. Boarding in a cattery or kennel, or a visit to the vet, can be extremely stressful, for both the unsocialised pet and the vet. Stressed animals are more susceptible to disease and many vets report longer recovery times after surgery or injury in fearful patients. Unsocialised cats and dogs are less likely to make rewarding pets and as a result may end up being abandoned, becoming strays or having to be re-homed. The subsequent cycle of multiple re-homings through animal shelters as each new owner in turn finds the animal unsuitable as a pet may eventually result in euthanasia or premature death.

Such problems are easily avoided if the right steps are taken early in the cat or dog's life. Although it is possible to accustom adult cats or dogs to new situations, this can be most easily achieved during the first 2 to 4 months of their life, before the fear reaction is fully established. A wide variety of experience in early life also has a priming effect on the ability of the animal to accept novel experiences and events later on in life. This is

why it is not essential for the breeder or owner of the puppy or kitten to anticipate every single stimulus that the animal will ever encounter. A wide range of representative experiences is all that is necessary in order to develop the animal's general ability to adapt to novel situations. A few simple steps, many of which are enjoyable in themselves for both the owner and the kitten or puppy, are usually all that is necessary to produce a well adjusted and rewarding pet.

The practical application of this idea will be expanded later in this chapter. First, it is necessary to examine the process by which the neonatal puppy or kitten becomes a fully functioning animal. This process is conventionally divided into several stages and it should always be borne in mind that the timing of these stages is not identical for cat and dog (Fig. 6.1).

Dog Socialisation

Behavioural Development in Dogs

The early development of the dog (and the wolf) can be divided into 4 distinct phases—the neonatal period, the transition period, the socialisation period and the juvenile period.[22,32,40,56] The neonatal and transition periods, which precede the development of social behaviour, are described by Nott[47] and will not be considered further here.

The socialisation period commences during the fourth week and lasts until the time at which bitches would, if left to their own devices, complete the weaning process (8–10 weeks). Play fighting begins at the beginning of this period and the puppies quickly learn to regulate the level of pain inflicted on their littermates, by reacting to distress vocalisations and then learning to inhibit their biting. By 4–5 weeks, the puppies begin to react specifically to the behaviour of their littermates, for example one puppy following another that has an object in its mouth. Facial expressiveness and aggressive vocalisations appear at about 5 weeks. Rapid maturation of motor patterns continues with the ability to run, climb and chew developing between 4 and 6 weeks. Between 3 and 5 weeks of age puppies readily approach novel stimuli, including unfamiliar people and dogs. Strong avoidance behaviour in response to unpleasant experiences develops thereafter and by 8 weeks a fear reaction can be expressed towards aversive stimuli.

By 6 weeks, most of the species-characteristic behaviour patterns can be observed. Fragments of sexual behaviour including mounting, clasping and pelvic thrusts may also be seen, especially in males. The level of fighting increases throughout the socialisation period with group attacks on one littermate occurring by 8–9 weeks. This is also the time when the first dominance hierarchies are formed, although these are not yet fixed.[7] It is during the socialisation period that a puppy is usually taken from its littermates and moved to another home. This homing should ideally be permanent since puppies frequently re-homed as juveniles seem more prone to behaviour problems in adulthood.[12,31]

Following the socialisation period is the juvenile period which lasts until sexual maturity, the end of the period varying enormously between particular breeds of dog. Food begging increases up to 16 weeks of age and dominance and submission signalling become well developed. Raised-leg urination in males appears between 5 and 8 months as does scratching after defecation. The level of imitative behaviour also increases.

Sensitive Periods

Most research into canine behavioural development has focused on the socialisation period because that is when a 'sensitive period' exists for bonding to people. This 'sensitive period' is an age range during which certain events are especially likely to have long term effects on an individual's development.[2] After this period, the individual gradually develops a lower sensitivity to those events. The term 'critical period', used in earlier studies of socialisation, implied a sharp cut-off in sensitivity unlike the gradual transition inherent in the concept of the 'sensitive period'.

The existence of a 'sensitive period' in canine development was first suggested by Scott and Marston[56] who followed the development of numerous puppies over several years. The biggest change in the relationship of puppies with their handlers occurred between 5 and 7 weeks of age, i.e. near the middle of the socialisation period. In timidity/confidence tests, the biggest change in reaction occurred at 5–6 weeks, again during the socialisation period. Scott and Marston[56] also proposed two other possible 'sensitive periods' for the dog, one immediately following birth, when the relationship with the dam is established and the other at the onset of sexual maturity. They suggested that all such periods may be of importance in the study of abnormal behaviour

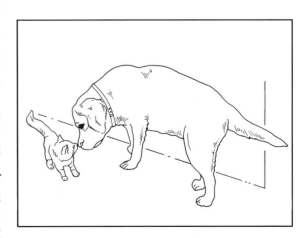

FIG. 6.2: Kittens can easily be socialised to dogs if they in turn are accepting of cats.

since 'traumatic experiences will have most effect during the critical periods'.

Puppies receiving only minimal human contact (e.g. just for feeding and cleaning) for their first 3–4 months often remain timid for the rest of their lives, particularly towards unfamiliar people, although there can be considerable variation, even within a single litter.[17] Observations of this kind have prompted detailed studies of socialisation in the dog and have revealed that socialisation with man takes place most readily between 3 and 12 weeks, with the optimum period being between 6 and 8 weeks.[25] In one study, bitches were allowed to raise their litters of puppies in a field with no human contact.[25] At varying ages, the puppies were removed from the field and given some socialisation with people, before being returned to their mother. All the animals were then tested for their level of attraction to humans at 14 weeks of age. Those socialised at 2–3 weeks scored low in the attraction test, those socialised at 5 weeks showed maximum attraction to the handler and those socialised at 9 weeks displayed a tendency to avoid the handler. The control group consisted of puppies which had remained in the field for the full 14 weeks with no socialisation at all. When tested for their level of attraction, these control puppies were extremely fearful and largely untrainable. Thus, if a dog has not had any experience of people by the age of 14 weeks, it becomes difficult to socialise and may remain essentially wild.

Quite brief experiences of social contact or isolation can induce changes in behaviour towards people, particularly if they occur towards the beginning of the socialisation period. In one study, the behaviour of puppies handled for 20 minutes each day between birth and 5 weeks was compared with puppies socially isolated for just the fifth week.[23] At 5 weeks of age, the handled puppies were more attracted to humans and in group tests they were dominant over the non-handled puppies. The isolated puppies were hyperactive in the presence of novel objects and tended to ignore their littermates in favour of self-play, or their physical surroundings. In general, they behaved similarly to puppies reared in social isolation for much longer than a week, the only difference being the lack of an avoidance response.

Puppies can become over-dependent on people if access to other dogs is prevented from 8 weeks of age. Such puppies tend to become asocial and may show aggression as a response to their fear of other dogs. Fox and Stelzner[24] compared groups of puppies hand-reared from several ages to determine effects of restricted socialisation to their own species. Puppies taken from their mothers at 3 days were aggressive towards other puppies when tested at 5, 8 and 12 weeks of age and tended to become temporarily dominant when the litters were reconstituted. Only puppies raised as litters for the first 8 weeks preferred canine to human company and initiated non-aggressive play with other puppies.

Most canine developmental research was carried out on beagles in highly restricted laboratory situations.[21,32] The value of extending these experimental results to dogs living as pets in a family home is questionable, especially given that one study claimed the amount of social experience required for puppies to behave like normal dogs is just 20 minutes per week,[26] which most authorities would consider to be far from adequate for a dog that is to become a pet. The beagle is commonly used as an experimental animal because it is both physically and temperamentally adaptable to an impoverished environment. Perhaps if breeds more representative of the general dog population had been used, different results might have been obtained, both in the timing of the different changes in behaviour and in the quality and quantity of stimuli required to trigger them. The process of socialisation is not rigid: taken as a whole, the scientific studies of early handling show that socialisation can vary greatly in terms of how it is conducted, how long is necessary and what styles are most effective and yet still result in the development of friendly dogs and cats. Practical considerations arising from this will be discussed later in the chapter.

Cat Socialisation

Behavioural Development in Cats

Socialisation is less well understood in the cat than in the dog. The four phases of behavioural development demonstrated in dogs, have not been experimentally derived in cats. However, the timings of different aspects of behavioural development have been summarised from several studies[52] and can be divided into at least 3 stages: the neonatal period; the socialisation period; and the juvenile period. The last two of these are important to the development of the cat–human relationship.

The socialisation period lies between the end of the second and seventh weeks and therefore starts earlier and ends earlier than the equivalent period in dogs. During this period, the time spent suckling decreases and kittens increasingly spend time actively exploring and learning about their environment.[52] Play increases and becomes more co-ordinated. Motor skills and sensory abilities develop rapidly. Weaning usually takes place during the socialisation period as kittens start to consume solid food.

The juvenile period is a term describing the period from the end of the 'sensitive period' for socialisation to people until the onset of sexual maturity. Kittens of this age are typically very playful and continue to develop their motor and sensory abilities. Although considerable variation exists, most kittens show signs of sexual maturity by 7 months of age. Oriental breeds are generally considered to mature earlier than average and pedigree long-haired breeds tend to be later than average.[19]

Sensitive Periods

Like puppies, kittens need to be handled if they are to develop into friendly, well-adjusted cats. Kittens have a 'sensitive period' for their socialisation to people, equivalent to that already described for puppies. After 7 weeks of age, socialisation has less of an effect on a cat's subsequent friendliness to people.[34] Cats handled between 1 and 5, 2 and 6, 3 and 7, or 4 and 8 weeks of age were compared for their response to people. Kittens remained longer with a test person and were most sociable if they had been handled between 2 and 6 weeks or 3 and 7 weeks of age. These kittens were more sociable than kittens handled for 4-week periods starting in the first week or ending in the eighth week.

Several studies have shown that even within the 'sensitive period', socialisation and subsequent attachment of the cat to its owner depends on many different aspects of early handling. The amount of handling, who handles the kitten, the style of handling and the presence of the queen, all influence its level of friendliness towards people.

Interacting with the litter in the presence of the queen seems to promote socialisation. If the queen is present her kittens are quicker to explore but more hesitant and cautious in her absence.[54] The mother's presence makes a strange situation more familiar for the kittens and enables them to encounter and learn about new things in a less threatening situation.[51] Kittens are also more confident if accompanied by their siblings[45] so are best socialised with their littermates. Some kittens will suffer from separation anxiety if their mother is absent even if they have their siblings around for company.

From studies in which the amount of handling that kittens received was varied, it is apparent that up to a certain limit, the more handling a kitten receives during the 'sensitive period', the friendlier it is likely to be.[33] Kittens handled for 40 minutes per day were friendlier to people than those handled for 15 minutes per day; they approached sooner and remained held for longer before attempting to escape. However, extending the amount of handling beyond an hour a day may produce little additional benefit. In a study of 9 litters of kittens born in homes, Bradshaw and Cook[6] found that litters handled for about 5 hours per day by their owners and their families were not consistently friendlier than litters handled for slightly less than 1 hour per day.

The relevance of the handler's relationship to the kitten for socialisation is still unknown. As the queen's behaviour influences the behaviour of her kittens,[11] her relationship with the handler may be important. If she is friendly with the handler, it is possible that this may promote her kittens' friendliness. Early experience of a wide range of people also helps a cat to be relaxed with people later in life. For example, kittens handled by 5 people were less fearful of an unknown person than were kittens handled by just a single person.[13] However, the kittens with a single handler showed more affectionate behaviour towards their handler than did the kittens with several handlers.

Certain styles of handling seem to be more effective than others at promoting friendliness in kittens. Evidence exists that exposure of young animals from several species to experiences that seem likely to be mildly aversive has beneficial effects on their ability to cope with stress later in life and on their rate of development and learning ability.[41,42,50] Animals can discriminate between styles of handling, so not all contact represents an equal stressor.[30] Food treats offered to the queen may help to calm and reassure her that the handler is not a threat to her litter and will increase attachment to the handler.[63] Speaking to cats while stroking them is a style of handling which favours their socialisation to people.[46] However, some cats prefer physical contact with their owners while others are more object orientated and prefer playing with their owners using toys.[61]

Guidelines for optimal socialisation are included in the later section on practical considerations.

The Effects of Domestication

The history of the dog's domestication is more clearly understood than the cat. Much of the dog's behaviour clearly has its origins in the behaviour of its ancestral species, the wolf, *Canis lupus*. The ancestor of the domestic cat is the African wild cat, *Felis silvestris lybica*[49] with a possible contribution from the Indian desert cat, *Felis silvestris ornata*, for the oriental breeds.[35] The cat is more recently domesticated than the dog and also seems more genetically resistant to the extreme modification that is evident in dogs from the enormous range in form and behaviour across breeds.[53] Feral dogs are rarely able to survive without some provisioning from people. In contrast, feral cats are still equipped to survive independently of people and can thrive on uninhabited islands.

Comparisons between the dog and wolf show that domestication has profoundly altered the characteristics of the socialisation period. During this period, many wolf puppies have a tendency to flee from man, whereas dog puppies will almost invariably approach people. Furthermore and more significantly, European wolves can only be socialised fully if they are removed from their dams before they are 2 weeks old and hand-reared,[66] although it is claimed that American wolves can be left with their dams somewhat longer before socialisation is inhibited.[65] This may be due to an inhibitory effect of a larger animal of the same species.[66] The wolf pup appears to have a well-defined 'template' which enables it to recognise its mother as the most appropriate object for attachment. If the wolf pup is removed from its mother, no such object is available and the template presumably broadens to the point that man becomes an effective substitute.

The ease with which domestic puppies and kittens can be socialised to a wide range of mammals (sheep, rabbits and cats, have all been successfully used as models for socialization), indicates that their 'template' is never as narrow as that of the wolf. This template favours attachment to conspecifics but extends to other species. For example, 4-week-old puppies that had been housed with a rabbit for as little as 24 hours exhibited a distress reaction when the rabbit was removed.[10] Likewise, kittens raised with Chihuahua puppies show distress when separated and are calmed when joined by one of the puppies. However, kittens raised with both kittens and a pup remain distressed when joined by the pup and only calm when joined by a kitten.[37] Chihuahua puppies raised by cat foster-mothers for a slightly longer period (from 25 days to 16 weeks) and then returned to their litters, were initially timid and acted submissively, but 2 weeks later they were displaying species-typical play behaviour.[20] Preferences for sexual partners do not appear to be established during the socialisation period, since the puppies raised with rabbits from 4 to 12 weeks of age and then reunited with their littermates, showed normal sexual preferences at one year.

Such experiments indicate the very adaptable nature of the puppy and kitten during their socialisation period; a wide range of mammalian models can be accepted as if they were members of the same species and even a mirror or a soft toy will reduce the level of distress vocalisation in a pup separated from its mother.[48] It appears that at this early stage in their life there is nothing particularly special about the initiation of their relationship with a person. At this age they are normally given the opportunity to bond to man, but can also form attachments to other mammals if available. Of course, the subsequent development of the relationship will differ greatly according to whether or not the partner is human.

Attachment

During socialisation the puppy or kitten learns its species identity which as indicated earlier, can be multiple.[20,36,37] From then on it will tend to direct its species-typical behaviour patterns, particularly communicative patterns, towards animals which match this identity. Other animals or people may induce a fear reaction, components of predatory behaviour, or a combination of both.

In a species as highly social as the dog, attachment behaviour is essential for maintaining social contacts and bonds between parent and offspring. Puppies react to separation from their mother and littermates by vocalising and increasing their activity level. Emotional reactions such as distress vocalisations are thought to be caused initially by distress due to absence of the familiar and then later by an associated fear of the unfamiliar. These two factors are compatible with each other and produce an additive effect.[58] As already described, queens and kittens, when separated, will also vocalise to remain in contact.

Vocalisation almost certainly accompanies internal distress. When a puppy or kitten is separated from familiar objects or locations, it vocalises to attract the attention of the parents or care-giving adults. These respond by seeking out their offspring and relieving their distress, hence reinforcing the social attachment.[55] Once the puppy or kitten has been weaned and is removed from the litter, its social attachment can shift to the human owner.[5] Separation problems (e.g. destruction, inappropriate elimination) are likely to occur, particularly in puppies, until they learn to tolerate some degree of social isolation.

What is required for an attachment to develop between a dog or cat and a person? Perhaps surprisingly, most experimental work has tended to indicate that attachment largely develops under mild stress, caused by separation or unfamiliar stimuli. For example, it has been suggested that handling is a beneficial form of stress, which if repeated over a period of time produces a more adaptable, less easily distressed animal.[23] Other kinds of stress also appear to stimulate attachment. Puppies reared with punishment as their only form of human contact were still attracted to people once the punishment had ceased.[18] Negative experiences therefore do not entirely inhibit the formation of an attachment. An increase in emotional reactions during the 'sensitive period' may bring about a higher level of dependency; for example, the process of socialisation to man can be speeded up by separating young puppies from their mother and placing them in a strange pen for 20 hours per day.[57] However, the consequences of such extreme manipulations for the behaviour of these dogs when adult were never recorded and these studies should not be used to support the use of punishment (negative reinforcement) as a training method.

A mechanism for attachment requires the following conditions:[58]

(i) The development of a memory of a stimulus previously experienced—a process of familiarisation.
(ii) The ability to discriminate the familiar from the unfamiliar.
(iii) The reaction of emotional distress in response to separation from the familiar.

The last-mentioned is the most controversial part of this model, since it suggests that attachment is driven by the negative reinforcement of separation from the attachment figure. It should not be thought, however, that welfare is necessarily impaired in this way. In the wolf and other wild carnivores, periodic absence of the mother for the purpose of hunting will occur as a natural part of a young animal's experience and the attachment mechanism may operate because of, rather than despite these absences and reunions.

Forty years ago it was thought that attachments were largely driven by the reward of food but Brodbeck[9] showed that feeding is not essential for attachment to develop. He eliminated the human–food association during the socialisation period, by feeding half his puppies himself and half mechanically. At other times, both groups were given equal amounts of human contact. At the end of the socialisation period both sets of puppies were equally attracted to the handler. Nor is food essential for attachment; indeed a degree of hunger seems to speed up the process. Elliot and King[15] hand fed a group of puppies, continually underfeeding some and constantly overfeeding others. It appeared that the underfed puppies were subsequently more attracted to the handler. However, the long-term consequences of underfeeding on behaviour were not recorded. More recently, a cat study showed that feeding can enhance the establishment of a relationship but is not sufficient to maintain it.[27] An outdoor cat colony was fed by a caretaker. For 11 days, two people unknown to the cats entered the enclosure after feeding had finished. Observation of cat response showed that one person was consistently preferred by the cats. During the experimental phase, the non-preferred person fed the cats without interacting with them, immediately left the enclosure and as before, returned with the second person only after feeding was finished. During the first half of the experimental phase, the new feeder became somewhat preferred, but neither person was preferred during the latter half. Geering[27] concluded that other interactions are required to cement a relationship such as petting, playing and vocalising.

Attachment can undoubtedly change after the end of the socialisation period, but little research has been carried out on this. Certain situations, including handrearing and early weaning, seem to contribute towards over-attachment to people during adolescence and later. Puppies removed from the litter before the socialisation period often lack the ability to interact normally with other dogs. Moreover, a dog that has not had any opportunity to play with others of its own species will tend to become too orientated towards humans.[32] Early attachment deprivation may also lead to an over-attachment developing later.[4] Such conditions are most likely to occur if puppies are given little human contact until they are 4–5 months old. This can occur in some pet shops, or in the increasing number of puppy farms.[28]

Changes in attachment between kittens and their owners undoubtedly occur during the first year of life, but very little systematic information has been collected in this area. Bradshaw and Smart[8] found that kittens between 3–5 months old had less than half the amount of interaction with their owners if they had been homed as a sibling pair than if they were the only kitten in the household. However, they were unable to determine whether the main factor determining this difference was the behaviour of the cats or the attitudes of the owners. Individual cats may also change dramatically in the way they react to being handled during the first 2 years of their lives.[6]

One problem in studying the causes of failures of attachment in adolescence and adulthood is that individual dogs or cats raised under similar conditions may react very differently to changes in their social environment. Senay[60] raised a litter of German Shepherd Dogs from 6 weeks to 9 months of age, allowing them little contact with other people or dogs. He was then absent for 2 months, during which time they received routine care only. During this period there was a considerable difference in the way the dogs reacted to being deprived of his company; the more confident individuals increased their object-seeking behaviour, whereas the more timid either avoided their new handler or became aggressive. The most plausible explanation for such differences is that they are related to dominance relationships between littermates. Dominance in social situations, boldness towards unfamiliar objects and fear of strange humans were all correlated in a litter of 5 male wolves, from about 10 weeks of age until at least 6 months.[39] 'Personalities' in both dogs and wolves are intrinsically unstable until the third month of life[7] which accounts for the unreliability of the Campbell puppy test which claims to predict adult behaviour when conducted at 7 weeks of age,[3] although fearfulness does show some stability.[29] These observations suggest that the juvenile period may contain a second 'sensitive period' for the further development of the dog's social attachments, but as yet scientific evidence is lacking.

Practical Considerations

Relationships between pets and people do not evolve within a vacuum. Puppies or kittens are open to an enormous array of new experiences which they must analyse, categorise and place in context. Basically, the wider their range of experience at this enormously impressionable stage, the better adjusted they will be to unexpected, startling and frightening events later in life. One model describes fear as the difference between what is expected by the animal and what it actually experiences.[1] A restricted early environment results in a large discrepancy and produces a timid pet which may be routinely aggressive or defensive because of fear of the unfamiliar.[32,59] To cite a specific case, 8 cats were brought into an animal shelter from a household where they had been confined in cattery-style accommodation. All of these cats habituated faster than expected to the observation cages in which the shelter placed cats for 24 hours after entry. They were soon behaving as normally-reared cats do: being friendly when approached or petted, grooming, feeding, defecating, urinating, moving about the cage and taking an interest in what was going on around them. However, when these cats were re-homed, all were returned because of disturbed behaviour. It seems the discrepancy between what they expected and what they observed was greater in their new homes than in the shelter cages. These cats were eventually successfully homed with people who initially caged them in one room, before gradually extending the area (and therefore variation) to which the cats had access.[43]

Puppies

Although puppies are born with only some of their sensory systems functioning, it should not be assumed that they are incapable of learning about their surroundings. Even new-born puppies can benefit from short periods of gentle handling. At this stage they pay a great deal of attention to the olfactory characteristics of their environment, so they can be made aware of the owner if pieces of cloth that have been previously handled, or (preferably) worn, are placed in the nest. These two experiences can be combined by holding the puppy close to the body while it is being handled.

As vision and hearing become functional during the transition phase, the range of stimuli to which the puppy can respond increases. Toys and other novel objects can be introduced even before the puppies are old enough to manipulate them. If the surroundings are generally quiet, a radio tuned to a station broadcasting programmes that include voices and natural sounds can be used to introduce variety. Alternatively, tapes of sound-effects can be played, although it should be remembered that a dog's hearing extends far into the ultrasound region, which radios and tapes do not reproduce. The amount of handling can be extended and a very soft brush can be used as a precursor to grooming. If the puppies' new owners have been decided at this stage, cloths that they have handled can also be introduced into the olfactory environment, to reduce the unfamiliarity of rehoming.

It is during the socialisation period that the greatest benefit can be gained from appropriate enrichment of the puppy's environment. Both socialisation (to people and other animals) and habituation (to inanimate stimuli) proceed side-by-side. If possible, the litter should be moved to a busy part of the house and kept in a wire-fronted enclosure to maximise their exposure to everyday occurrences. The enclosure should incorporate a secluded sleeping area to allow the puppies to withdraw when they wish to do so. From the security of this enclosure they should be introduced to as wide a range of people, including children, as is practicable. Any cats in the household will probably take this opportunity to investigate the puppies, providing them with another useful experience. Once socialisation is in progress, each puppy should be separated from its littermates and mother for short periods and eventually should be isolated completely for a few moments at a time. This will provide training in the idea that separations are followed by reunions and should lead to a dog better able to cope with spending time on its own later on in life. The puppy should be allowed to walk on as wide a variety of surfaces as possible; many

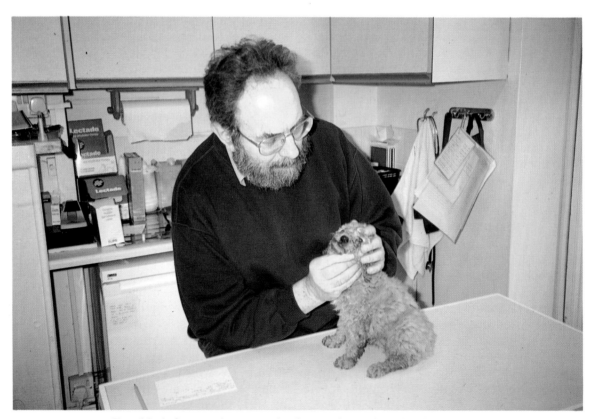

FIG. 6.3: A first veterinary examination can be made easier if the puppy has been previously placed on a table and stroked.

puppies arrive at their new homes thinking that the whole world is covered in newspaper! Handling can be extended to include games and more extended grooming. The beneficial effects of temporary mild stress can be achieved by picking up each puppy in turn and holding it in mid-air until it begins to protest, then holding it in contact with the body and stroking it until it is relaxed again. It may also be beneficial to place and then stroke the puppy on a table, as preparation for its first visit to the vet.

Re-homing should normally take place at between 6 and 8 weeks of age, i.e. in the middle of the socialisation period. This allows the puppy to re-establish its social environment in its new home, before its fear reaction to novel stimuli has developed. The transition can be made as smooth as possible by minimising the discontinuities between the environments provided by the breeder and the new owner. Transfer of scents, as described above, is likely to be more effective than may be imagined, given that dogs rely much more on olfactory information than do humans. However, during the socialisation period there is probably no substitute for actual encounters with the new owner while the puppy is still with the breeder. After re-homing, the process described above should be continued, well into the juvenile period.

Kittens

Many of the principles described for puppies are also appropriate for kittens. Like puppies, the general approach is to start introducing variation at an early age, both social (people and other animals) and environmental (radios, a busy location in the house, etc.) At 2 weeks of age, gentle handling should begin for short periods of just a few minutes. The kittens should be spoken to while being stroked. The length of the sessions should gradually increase and start to include less familiar people, eventually including visitors to the house whom they have not previously encountered.

Kittens should initially be handled in the presence of the queen. If the queen is nervous, the sessions should be limited to about 1 minute at first and she should be constantly reassured by gentle speaking and then stroking. It may also be useful to adopt a less threatening posture by getting down to the same level as the queen. Once the queen is reasonably relaxed the kittens can be handled.

Many cats are very particular about which part of their body is stroked, only just tolerating or responding aggressively to certain areas being touched; usually the underbelly and sides of the abdomen. However, kittens should at first be touched on all parts of their body and frequently lifted and gently restrained so they become accustomed to being handled.

Toys can be introduced as soon as the kittens have had some experience of people. As they develop, it becomes apparent that some kittens prefer physical contact with their owners while others are more object orientated and prefer interacting with their owners by playing with toys. The variety and complexity of the toys and household items which the kitten experiences should gradually increase over time.

Many non-pedigree kittens move to their new home at about 6–8 weeks of age. At present, the optimal age for homing has not been established but breeders tend to home

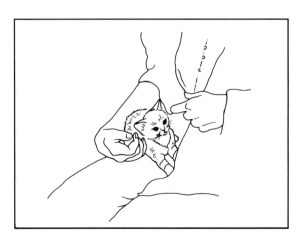

FIG. 6.4: Gentle handling of kittens for a few minutes each day should begin at 2 weeks of age.

pedigree kittens a little later, usually around 12 weeks of age. Therefore, most kittens will, at best, be reaching the end of their peak socialisation period when they move. Consequently, the responsibility for starting a sensitive and imaginative socialisation programme falls on the breeder, especially if the kittens are not to be homed until 12 weeks of age. The new owner's responsibility is to continue this programme well into the juvenile period.

Social Referencing

Fear of the unfamiliar can be further minimised by introducing puppies and kittens to an even wider variety of situations during their juvenile periods. Dog trainers often refer to this process as 'socialisation', a term which should strictly speaking be restricted to the primary (species) socialisation period, as defined in this chapter. To avoid confusion, we propose the term **social referencing** to refer to the broadening of the animal's experience during the juvenile period.

Puppy trainers have learned by experience that social referencing is achieved much more easily if the puppy is under 14 weeks of age. Likewise, if kittens are not handled or exposed to variety within their first 12 weeks they rarely become friendly or relaxed cats. Unfortunately some vaccination regimes make it difficult to present the young animal with a wide range of experiences during the first 12 weeks. The puppy or kitten is vulnerable to infection when protection from maternal antibodies has decreased to inadequate levels but has yet to complete its early vaccination programme. Thus, schemes which give protection from about 6 weeks are preferable for achieving social referencing.

It is also possible to broaden the experience of kittens and puppies, without exposing them to infection, by carrying them about in a travelling box. Novel experiences can be presented in the home, either as they arise (e.g. careful introductions to human visitors) or deliberately (puppies and kittens are often taken in by simple disguises such as hats,

wigs and false beards). Socialisation classes for puppies are available in some countries; they provide a wealth of valuable experience and can be managed in such a way that puppies which have had their first vaccinations are exposed to minimal risk of infection. It is often forgotten that kittens need to learn about other cats as their social life is rarely restricted to their home. Other cats in the household can teach kittens not just about the unpredictability of their environment but also cat–cat social skills.

The following checklist suggests some experiences which should benefit a puppy. Although much less is known about the factors that can reduce timidity in cats, some of these may also be effective for kittens.

- People who differ from those encountered in the animal's home. Whenever possible this should include people of both sexes, a variety of ages, and people from differing ethnic groups. People of differing appearance from those encountered in the animal's home, such as individuals with or without beards and/or spectacles, and people who may visit the home in some form of uniform (e.g. postal delivery personnel, refuse collectors, and policemen) should also be encountered. An individual's appearance may be modified by other objects and so young animals should be exposed to people carrying rucksacks, sacks or boxes, people in wheelchairs or on crutches, and to children in pushchairs.
- People in groups in order to introduce the animal to noise and activity e.g. groups of children in a playground.
- Fast-moving people, who may trigger a predatory (chasing) response e.g. joggers, cyclists, people on skateboards or rollerskates.
- Animals, including friendly dogs of different sizes and appearances, long-haired, large and flat faced dogs, cats, livestock.
- Different environments e.g. travelling in cars, buses, trains, underground trains, lifts and escalators, walking near traffic and on different types of surface.

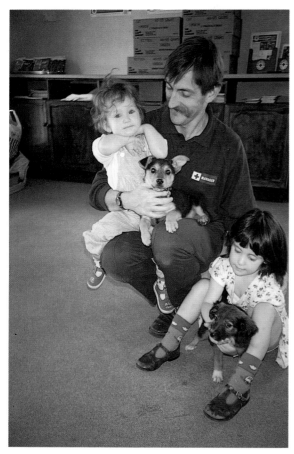

FIG. 6.5: Supervised contact beween puppies and children will provide valuable experience for both parties.

Since urban dogs are likely to be taken for occasional walks in the countryside, and most rural dogs will visit towns from time to time, some early experience of both environments is likely to prove valuable.

Methods of training puppies in the acceptance of novel situations have changed dramatically over the years and now de-emphasise punishment, bringing improvements both to the puppy's welfare and to the long-term effectiveness of the training. Positive reinforcement (e.g. patting or giving a food reward) whenever the puppy reacts neutrally to a novel stimulus has proved to be the best way of achieving a confident personality. Rewards such as stroking or patting following fearful or aggressive reactions simply serve to reinforce those reactions and are counterproductive, as is punishment under the same circumstances. Fearful responses by the dog towards specific people or objects can often be reduced by the owner making a positive response towards the target of the fear. The puppy should then react to the social cues that the owner is providing and become curious rather than frightened. This approach is worth adopting even if its application can appear bizarre. To quote one case, a puppy that was frightened of metal dustbins was cured by the owner ignoring the puppy while talking to and patting a dustbin!

Heritable Effects

Genetic differences in behaviour interact with the effects of socialisation, driving the development of temperament in puppies or kittens. Most of the handling studies have not controlled for genetic differences in temperament, although some authors have suggested a genetic origin for individual differences in kittens handled to the same degree.[33,46] Turner et al.[62] could distinguish kittens in a laboratory colony by the friendliness of their father, a genetically mediated effect as the kittens had never seen their father. McCune[41] has examined how this genetic effect interacts with early handling. Father's friendliness and early handling had an additive effect; the friendliest kittens had been socialised and came from the friendlier of two fathers. The genetic component of friendliness was reinterpreted as 'boldness', because identity of the father differentiated kittens not only in their response to people but also to a novel object. The benefit to these kittens of being bolder was seen when they were introduced to strangers and when caged for 24 hours. Compared to kittens from the unfriendly father they were less distressed, showed less inhibition of normal behaviour and habituated sooner.[42] In pet kittens, this heritable tendency towards boldness appears to persist until at least the end of the first year.[6] Another recent study has demonstrated paternal effects for socialisation/friendliness and reactivity/aggression using 5 fathers.[50] Ledger[38] also detected a genetic basis for differences between kittens of pedigree British Shorthair cats in their response to people. She found that kittens carrying the gene for red coat colour were more difficult to handle and made more escape attempts from people in a holding test.

As differences between individuals in their response to people and to novelty can be explained in part by heritable factors, breeders should breed from dogs and cats that are confident and friendly with people.[16,41] Since the quantitative estimation of the heritability of temperament is still in its infancy, this can only be carried out on a qualitative basis at present and may therefore carry an element of luck.[64] Selection for good temperament in pedigree breeds can only be successful if two conditions are satisfied: heritability must be high, and sufficient variability in the genetic basis for temperament must be present in the breed. If we still know little about how to select for desirable behaviour in pedigree animals, we can be even less precise about the heritability of temperament in mongrel dogs and cats.

We can be much more certain about the right environment in which to raise a puppy or kitten than we can about the design of breeding programmes to improve temperament. Thus, the provision of a suitable environment and socialisation programme is vital to the appropriate development of our companion animals.

References

1. Archer, J. (1979) Behavioural aspects of fear. In *Fear in Animals and Man.* Ed. W. Sluckin, pp. 56–85. Van Nostrand Reinhold, New York.
2. Bateson, P. (1979) How do sensitive periods arise and what are they for? *Animal Behaviour,* **27,** 470–486.
3. Beaudet, R. and Dallaire, A. (1993) Social dominance evaluation: observations on Campbell's test. *Bulletin on Veterinary Clinical Ethology,* **1,** 23–29.
4. Borchelt, P. L. (1983) Separation elicited behavior problems in dogs. In *New Perspectives on our Lives with Companion Animals.* Eds. A. H. Katcher and A. M. Beck. pp. 187–196. University of Pensylvannia Press, Philadelphia.
5. Borchelt, P. L. and Voith, V. L. (1982) Diagnosis and treatment of separation-related behaviour problems in dogs. *Veterinary Clinics of North America (Small Animal Practice),* **12,** 625–635.
6. Bradshaw, J. W. S. and Cook, S. E. Unpublished data
7. Bradshaw, J. W. S. and Nott, H. M. R. (in press) Social and communication behaviour of companion dogs. In *The Domestic Dog: its Evolution, Behaviour and Interactions with People.* Ed. J. A. Serpell. Cambridge University Press.
8. Bradshaw, J. W. S. and Smart, F. R. E. (1993) Behavioural differences between kittens homed singly and in pairs. *Journal of the Feline Advisory Bureau,* **30,** 141–143.
9. Brodbeck, A. (1954) An exploratory study on the acquisition of dependency behaviour in puppies. *Bulletin of the Ecological Society of America,* **35,** 73.
10. Cairns, R. B. and Werboff, J. (1967) Behaviour development in the dog: an interspecific analysis. *Science,* **158,** 1070–1072.
11. Chesler, P. (1969) Maternal influence in learning by observation in kittens. *Science,* **166,** 901–903.
12. Christians, A., Bradshaw, J. W. S. and Bailey, G. P. Unpublished data.
13. Collard, R. (1967) Fear of strangers and play behaviour in kittens with varied social experience. *Child Development,* **38,** 877–891.
14. Council for Science and Society Report (1988) In *Companion Animals in Society.* Oxford University Press.
15. Elliot, O. and King, J. A. (1960) The effect of early food deprivation on later consummatory behaviour in puppies. *Psychological Reports,* **6,** 391–400.
16. Fält, L. (1984) Inheritance of behaviour in the dog. In *Nutrition and Behaviour in Dogs and Cats.* Ed. R. S. Anderson. pp. 183–187. Pergamon Press, Oxford.
17. Feddersen-Petersen, D. (1993) Some interactive aspects between dogs and their owners: are there reciprocal influences between both inter- and intra-specific communication? In *Proceedings of the International Congress on Applied Ethology, Berlin.* Eds. M. Nichelmann, H. K. Wierenga and S. Braun. pp. 182–189. Humboldt University, Berlin.
18. Fisher, A. E. (1955) The effects of differential early treatment on the social and exploratory behaviour of puppies.'PhD Thesis, Pensylvannia State University.
19. Fogle, B. (1991) *The Cat's Mind.* Pelham Books, London.
20. Fox, M. W. (1969) Behavioral effects of rearing dogs with cats during the 'critical period of socialization'. *Behaviour,* **35,** 273–280.

21. Fox, M. W. (1978) *The Dog: its Domestication and Behaviour.* Garland STPM Press, New York.

22. Fox, M. W. and Bekoff, M. (1975) The behaviour of dogs. In *The Behaviour of Domestic Animals.* Ed. E. S. E. Hafez. pp. 370–409. Balliere, Tindall and Cox, London.

23. Fox, M. W. and Stelzner, D. (1966) Behavioural effects of differential early experience in the dog. *Animal Behaviour*, **14**, 273–281.

24. Fox, M. W. and Stelzner, D. (1967) The effects of early experience on the development of inter- and intraspecies social relationships in the dog. *Animal Behaviour*, **15**, 377–386.

25. Freedman, D., King, J. and Elliot O. (1961) Critical periods in the social development of dogs. *Science*, **133**, 1016–1017.

26. Fuller, J. (1964) Effects of experiential deprivation upon behaviour in animals. *Proceedings of the Third World Congress of Psychiatry.* University of Toronto Press.

27. Geering, K. (1986) Der Einfluss der Fütterung auf die Katze-Mensch-Beziehung. Thesis, Zoology Institute, University of Zurich-Irchel.

28. Goddard, M. (1993) Separation anxiety. In *The Behaviour of Dogs and Cats.* Ed. J. Fisher. pp. 62–75. Stanley Paul and Co. Ltd, London.

29. Goddard, M. E. and Beilharz, R. G. (1986) Early prediction of adult behaviour in potential guide dogs. *Applied Animal Behaviour Science*, **15**, 247–260.

30. Hemsworth, P. H., Barnett, J. L. and Hansen, C. (1986) The influence of handling by humans on the behaviour, reproduction and corticosteroids of male and female pigs. *Applied Animal Behaviour Science*, **15**, 303–314.

31. Houpt, K. A. (1985) Companion animal behaviour: a review of dog and cat behaviour in the field, in the laboratory and the clinic. *Cornell Veterinarian*, **75**, 248–261.

32. Houpt, K. A. and Wolski, T. (1982) Development of behaviour. In *Domestic Animal Behaviour for Veterinarians and Animal Scientists.* Iowa State University Press.

33. Karsh, E. B. (1984) Factors influencing the socialization of cats to people. In *The Pet Connection: its Influence on our Health and Quality of Life.* Eds. R. K. Anderson, B. L. Hart, and L. A. Hart. pp. 207–215. University of Minnesota Press.

34. Karsh, E. B. and Turner, D. C. (1988) The human–cat relationship. In *The Domestic Cat: the Biology of its Behaviour.* Eds. D. C. Turner, and P. Bateson. pp. 159–177. Cambridge University Press.

35. Kratochvil, J. and Kratochvil, Z. (1976) The origin of the domestic forms of the genus *Felis* (*Mammalia*). *Zoologicke Listy*, **25**, 193–208.

36. Kuo, Z. Y. (1930) The genesis of the cat's response to the rat. *Journal of Comparative Psychology*, **11**, 1–35.

37. Kuo, Z. Y. (1960) Studies on the basic factors in animal fighting VII. Interspecies coexistence in mammals. *Journal of Genetic Psychology*, **97**, 211–225.

38. Ledger, R. (1993) Factors influencing responses of kittens to humans and novel objects. MSc Thesis, University of Edinburgh.

39. MacDonald, K. (1987) Development and stability of personality characteristics in pre-pubertal wolves: Implications for pack organization and behaviour. In *Man and Wolf.* Ed. H. Frank. Dr W Junk Publishers, Dordrecht.

40. Markwell, P. J. and Thorne, C. J. (1987) Early behavioural development of dogs. *Journal of Small Animal Practice*, **28**, 984–991.

41. McCune, S. (1992) Temperament and the welfare of caged cats. PhD Thesis, University of Cambridge.

42. McCune, S. (1994) Caged cats: avoiding problems and providing solutions. *Newsletter of the Companion Animal Behaviour Study Group*, No. 7.

43. McCune, S. (in press) Coping with confinement: temperament effects on how domestic cats adjust to caging and handlers. *Proceedings of the 1st Conference on Environmental Enrichment.* Portland.

44. Meier, G. W. and Stuart, J. L. (1959) Effects of handling on the physical and behavioural development of Siamese kittens. *Psychological Reports*, **5**, 497–501.

45. Mendl, M. (1986) Effects of litter size and sex of young on behavioural development in domestic cats. PhD Thesis, University of Cambridge.

46. Moelk, M. (1979) The development of friendly approach behaviour in the cat: a study of kitten–mother relations and the cognitive development of the kitten from birth to 8 weeks. *Advances in the Study of Behaviour*, **10**, 163–224

47. Nott, H. M. R. (1992) Social behaviour of the dog. In *The Waltham Book of Dog and Cat Behaviour.* Ed. C. Thorne. pp. 97–114. Pergamon Press, Oxford.

48. Pettijohn, T. F., Wong, T. W., Ebert, P. D. and Scott, J. P. (1977) Alleviation of separation distress in 3 breeds of young dogs. *Developmental Psychobiology*, **10**, 373–381.

49. Randi, E. and Ragni, B. (1991) Genetic variability and biochemical systematics of domestic and wild cat populations (*Felis silvestris: Felidae*). *Journal of Mammalogy*, **72**, 79–88.

50. Reisner, I. R., Houpt, K. A., Hollis, N. E. and Quimby, F. W. (1994) Friendliness to humans and defensive aggression in cats: the influence of handling and paternity. *Physiology and Behaviour*, **55**, 1119–1124.

51. Rheingold, H. and Eckermann, C. (1971) Familiar social and non-social stimuli and the kittens response to a strange environment. *Developmental Psychobiology*, **4**, 71–89. Cited in: Guyot, G. W., Cross, H. A. and Bennett, T. L. (1983) Early social isolation of the domestic cat: responses during mechanical toy testing. *Applied Animal Behaviour. Science*, **10**, 109–116.

52. Robinson, I. H. (1992) Behavioural development of the cat. In *The Waltham Book of Dog and Cat Behaviour*. Ed. C. Thorne. pp. 53–64. Pergamon Press, Oxford.

53. Robinson, R. (1984) Cat. In *Evolution of Domesticated Animals*. Ed. I. L. Mason. pp. 217–225 Longman, London.

54. Rodel, H. (1986) Faktoren, die den Aufbau einer Mensch-Katze-Beziehung beeinflussen. Thesis, Zoology Institute, University of Zurich-Irchel. Cited in: Karsh, E. B. and Turner, D. C. (1988) The Human–cat relationship. In *The Domestic Cat: The Biology of its Behaviour*. Eds. D. C. Turner and P. Bateson. pp. 159–177. Cambridge University Press.

55. Scott, J. P. (1967) The evolution of social behaviour in dogs and wolves. *American Zoologist*, **7**, 373–381.

56. Scott, J. P. and Marston, M. V. (1950) Critical periods affecting the development of normal and mal-adjustive social behaviour of puppies. *The Journal of Genetic Psychology*, **77**, 25–60.

57. Scott, J. P., Deshaies, D. and Morris, D. D. (1962) The effect of emotional arousal on primary socialization in the dog. Cited in: Scott and Fuller (1965) *Genetics and the Social Behaviour of the Dog*. Chicago University Press, Chicago.

58. Scott, J. P., Stewart, J. M. and DeGhett, V. J. (1973) Separation in infant dogs. In *'Separation and Depression' Clinical and Research Aspects*. Eds. J. P. Scott and E. C. Senay. pp. 3–32. American Association for the Advancement of Science Symposium.

59. Seitz, P. F. D. (1959) Infantile experience and adult behaviour in animal subjects. II Age of separation from the mother and adult behaviour in the cat. *Psychosomatic Medicine*, **21**, 353–378.

60. Senay, E. C. (1966) Toward an animal model of depression: a study of separation behaviour in dogs. *Journal of Psychiatric Research*, **4**, 65–71.

61. Turner, D. C. (1991) The ethology of the human–cat relationship. *Swiss Archive for Veterinary Medicine*, **133**, 63–70.

62. Turner, D. C., Feaver, J., Mendl, M. and Bateson, P. (1986) Variations in domestic cat behaviour towards humans: a paternal effect. *Animal Behaviour*, **34**, 1890–2.

63. Wenzel, B. M. (1959) Tactile stimulation as reinforcement for cats and its relation to early feeding experience. *Psychological Reports*, **5**, 297–300. Cited by: Fox, M. W. (1975) The behaviour of cats. In *The Behaviour of Domestic Animals*, 3rd edn. Eds. E. S. E. Hafez. pp. 410–436. Balliere, Tindall and Cox, London.

64. Willis, M. B. (1987) Breeding dogs for desirable traits. *Journal of Small Animal Practice*, **28**, 965–983.

65. Woolpy, J. H. and Ginsburg, B. E. (1967) Wolf socialization: a study of temperament in a wild social species. *American Zoologist*, **7**, 357–363.

66. Zimen, E. (1987) Ontogeny of approach and flight behaviour towards humans in wolves, poodles and wolf–poodle hybrids. In *Man and Wolf*. Ed. H. Frank. pp. 275–292. Dr W. Junk Publishers, Dordrecht.

CHAPTER 7

The Human–Cat Relationship

DENNIS C. TURNER

Introduction

Human–cat relationships have existed for several thousands of years although these relationships have been researched for only a relatively few years. However, from this recent information, a picture of factors affecting the content, structure and quality of these interspecific relationships is beginning to emerge. This chapter will attempt to integrate those findings and include thought-provoking ideas for future research.

Factors Affecting the Human–Cat Relationship

The character traits of today's two most popular companion species, cats and dogs, are very different. Potential owners are well advised to consider the adjectives used by experienced owners to describe each species before considering their desires, needs and ability to house the selected animal according to its own biological and psychological needs.[1,2,16,19–21] Dogs are often described as being rational, communicative, easily understood, obedient, faithful and protective; cats are considered to be irrational, erotic, loving,

elegant, natural, independent, stubborn, quicker to react, calming, quiet, cleaner and less expensive than their counterparts. Interestingly, although the cat, as a species, was originally thought to be solitary and anti-social, recent studies have shown that it is quite capable of becoming sociable.[3,8,9,21,24]

Experience of Humans

In the last chapter, the importance of socialising kittens with humans was stressed.[3,7] Later social behaviour towards both humans and conspecifics is more or less determined by events and experiences during this phase.[12,15,20] Tests are currently being developed to help determine the original socialisation status and optimal housing conditions for cats in animal shelters, therefore aiding the decision of future rehoming.

Other factors can also influence the development of the relationship between cats and humans.[7,15] The kitten–human relationship is affected by the type of relationship that the mother cat has with humans. Depending on her own social behaviour towards humans, she may or may not hide her litter. Consequently this affects the timing of their first contact with humans. Also, observations suggest that the presence or absence of the mother when the kittens have contact with humans can affect the relationship. The genetic history of the parents also impacts on kitten behaviour, although it is difficult to separate traits that may have been learnt from the mother from those that were inherited (*See* [15,23] and Chapter 6).

Animals not originally socialised with humans require a great deal of patience before they will accept their caretaker as a social partner. Usually these cats remain 'one person' or 'one family' cats, wary of all other people, especially when outside their home.[10] On the other hand, well socialised cats are easily able to establish contact with new human partners, even after negative experiences with other humans.[15] In both cases, it has been shown that it is important that the cat initiates the social contacts, rather than the human partner.[17,18] There are several ways in which the development and stability of the human–cat relationship can be affected.[15,16,20] The act of feeding the animal (irrespective of what is fed) has a positive effect on contact establishment. However, trials have also shown that feeding alone is insufficient to maintain the social bond; if the feeder does not respond to the cat's approaches by speaking, or stroking, the preference for contact with the feeding person disappears relatively quickly.[21]

Social relationships can be defined by the content, quality and temporal patterning of their component interactions[5,6] and there are many different kinds of interactions between humans and their cats. The diversity of inter-actions involved is important in that each partner in the relationship learns more about the behavioural style (the 'personality') of his or her counterpart by interacting in different situations. Obviously, a relationship that exhibits only feeding interactions (a so-called **'uniplex' relationship**) has a different content, quality and temporal patterning than one which exhibits feeding, play, stroking and vocal interactions (a **'multiplex' relationship**).

Early studies have shown that companion animals are most frequently found in households in which the adults experienced companion animals themselves as children and

usually it is the same species.[14] Since cats and dogs have different communicative signals, it is reasonable to expect that one feels most comfortable with the companion species one has learnt to 'understand'.

Individuality and Cat Character Traits

Domestic cats are well known for their 'individuality', a parameter so significant that it has had to be statistically considered in most studies.[7,11,13,18,21] Interacting with our own cats in different situations helps us learn the individual 'quirks' of our own animals and cement the relationships, making each relationship unique.

Often cats are selected simply on the basis of their appearance, in particular coat colour,[7] regardless of behavioural needs or character traits. For example, all kittens play, but not all adult cats; nor do all adult cats appreciate close physical contact or being stroked. Research has shown that most adult cats can be separated into those preferring to play and those preferring contact; but most people would like to have both characteristics in the same cat and might be disappointed if they are unaware of this.[13,17]

When selecting a cat, one also has to consider whether or not the cat is to be kept only indoors or allowed outside and whether one or more than one cat is desirable. In areas with heavy traffic, one might opt for indoor housing. In these cases, it is crucial that the cat selected has been raised indoors and that the home is furnished in order for the cat to be able to satisfy all of its biological and motivational needs (discussed later). For people living alone or couples where both partners work, indoor cats should not be kept alone. However, where more than one cat is kept, **all** cats living in the same primary home **must** have been socialised with other cats as kittens,[18] even if outdoor access is available. Cats are usually social with other cats if they stem from a large litter (4 or more) and have remained together with their littermates for at least 10, or preferably 12, weeks. Positive contact with other adult cats during this period can also aid sociability.[12]

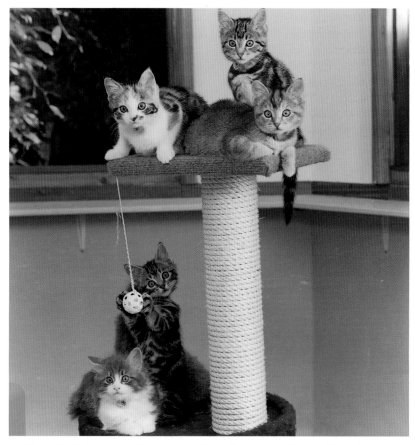

FIG. 7.1: Cats are usually social to others if they stem from a litter of four or more and have remained together with their littermates for 10 or 12 weeks.

Breed Differences

When selecting a cat, one is immediately faced with the question: pedigree or non-pedigree? Dogs have been domesticated and selectively bred for much longer than cats and have specific behavioural traits. Until recently, cats were bred only for appearance (body form, coat colour and hair characteristics) and rarely for behavioural traits. However, the consistency of cat breed descriptions leads one to believe that character differences exist between breeds. Recently the first ethological studies of behavioural differences between selected cat breeds were conducted and combined with cat character assessments made by their owners.[17,18,21,26] In the most recent study,[21] two of the oldest and reputedly

different breeds, the Siamese and Persian, were compared with non-pedigree cats and some interesting discoveries were made.

Some aspects of the general character descriptions were confirmed. In this study, Siamese were more playful, active, vocal and demonstrative than Persians. However, many more differences were found between the pedigree cats and the non-pedigree than between the two pedigree breeds themselves. Differences between the pedigree and non-pedigree cats were most often in favour of the pedigree cats, or the relationships with them. The pedigree cats appeared to be more friendly towards people providing (or allowing) more interaction time, longer interactions and closer contact. At the same time their owners rated them as being more predictable and less independent than the typical non-pedigree cat. All of these results speak for convergent selection during the development of the breeds, rather than divergent selection.[21] These results should not detract from the value of non-pedigree cats as pets. Many people are completely satisfied with a non-pedigree cat, they can make excellent companions and form the majority of the pet cat population.

Sex of the Cat

No significant differences in behaviour towards people have been found between male and female cats.[13] Most of the cats involved in such colony and household studies were either spayed or castrated, which may have masked any differences, if they existed. Nevertheless, most privately owned cats are also neutered and so these results are relevant to the general population. Two points should still be considered when selecting the sex of a companion cat. Intact males have much larger ranges than intact females and because of this, are often exposed to more danger (such as traffic), although neutering reduces range size.[3,9] As females have generally smaller ranges than males, it might be more appropriate to select a female if the cat is not going to be allowed outdoors.[12] Keeping intact females indoors during oestrus without access to males is not recommended; they show their restlessness with increased activity and noise and come into heat repeatedly. Unless there is an intention to breed from the cat, females should be neutered.

Sex and Age of the Person

A study was performed on cat and human behaviour during first encounters between cats and people unknown to them, when the humans were instructed not to intitiate interaction. The cats showed no preference for a particular age (adult versus child) or sex.[11,13,21] However, as soon as the human subjects

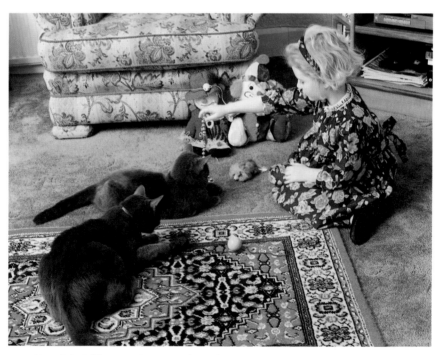

FIG. 7.2: Differences in a cat's behaviour towards an individual are caused by the way that individual interacts with the cat.

were allowed to interact, the cats showed statistical differences in their reactive behaviour depending on the age and sex of the human. Thus, it is the human who shows differences in behaviour towards the cat and the cat reacts differentially to that. In established relationships, learning will certainly also play an important role.

Men tend to interact while seated; women and girls move down to the level of the cat (on the floor) more often. Adults usually call the cats first, allowing the cat to do the approaching; children, especially boys, approach the cats directly, which is not always accepted by the animals. Women also speak to cats more frequently and tend to be the main interactional partner.[11] Women are also more frequently approached[11] by cats and the animals are generally more willing to cooperate with them than with men.[21]

Housing Conditions

Three housing factors have been analysed for a potential effect on cat behaviour and human attitudes. These are the number of humans in the household, the number of cats kept and whether or not the cats are allowed outdoors.[11,17,18,21] The smaller the human family, the more social attention the cat gives each member. Social play by the cat lasts longer and contact rubbing is shown more often in smaller families than in larger ones. Single cats spend significantly more time interacting with their owners than cats in multiple-cat households.[18] These differences were most often due to differences in the person's behaviour towards single cats and cats in multiple-cat households and not the cat's behaviour (e.g. amount of contact initiation). Qualitatively, it appears that owners pamper single cats, which is perhaps more difficult to do when several cats live together. Indeed, owners of multiple cats stated that they wished their cats would be less fussy about food more often than owners of single cats did; they were also somewhat less tolerant of their cat's curiosity, than owners of single animals.[17]

Several differences in interactional behaviour have been found between indoor cats and cats allowed outdoors. Indoor cats are generally more active but show less head/flank rubbing on their human partners than cats with outdoor access.[11] The latter do much more 'greeting' (rubbing) when they come home from an outdoor excursion. Taking differences in potential interaction time (time at home) into account, indoor cats spend more time interacting with their human partners (including more play and more time close to their partners) than outdoor cats do when they are at home. This is due to more contact initiation by the indoor cats and it has been suggested that they may be compensating for some lack of environmental stimuli indoors, relative to outdoors, by interacting more often with their human partners.[18] The person becomes an important source of stimulation for indoor cats. Owners of indoor and outdoor cats attach different importance to the human–cat relationship and show differing amounts of dissatisfaction in their cat's behaviour.[17] These differences help us understand a number of features of human–cat relationships. Owners of cats allowed outside wish that their animals were less friendly to strangers than do owners of indoor cats. Outdoor cats were also rated as being less curious than indoor cats, again suggesting that indoor cats actively seek out stimulation, either with objects or people.

Interestingly, owners of cats allowed outdoors rate their animals higher on measures of independence and also state that their cats **should be** more independent than do the owners of indoor cats. In contrast, owners of indoor cats often state that they wish their animals would remain close to them (within 1 metre). Thus, independence and frequent proximity to human partners are not necessarily compatible.[17]

Living in Harmony

Expectations of Cat Ownership

Turning to psychological aspects of the human–cat relationship, in one study over

150 cat owners were asked to rate their animals in terms of character traits (both positive and negative). The data were then analysed for positive and negative correlations between traits.[17] A high level of perceived affection towards the owner was positively associated with high affection by the owner towards the cat and both traits were positively associated with high ratings for cleanliness and predictability. High ratings on enjoyment of physical contact (by the cat) and proximity were also positively associated with perceived affection towards the human partner.

The negative correlations between traits are equally interesting.[17] The owner's affection towards the animal was rated higher the less often urine-spraying occurred in the house and the less restless the cat was at night. Cats rated as being restless at night were also judged to be less predictable and these, in turn, were rated higher on aggressiveness

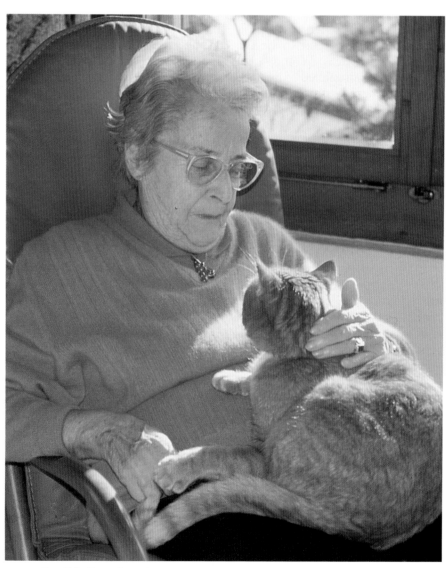

FIG. 7.3: Cats who enjoy physical contact are perceived as being affectionate by their owners. © I.E.T./I.E.A.P.

towards their owners. Cats which were restless at night were also considered to be less affectionate towards their owners. Interestingly, humans associate feline independence with lower affection towards themselves and the more independent the cat, the lower its 'likeness to humans' was rated.

One aspect of the human–cat relationship has received little attention to date, namely, the strength of bond with the cat and how that influences the relationship. There is some evidence that the strength of bond affects rehoming of cats adopted from a shelter.[7] The stronger the bond to the cat, the less likely it is that the owner will subsequently try to rehome it. Since a relatively large number of animals are rehomed from shelters each year, more work in this area is needed to predict outcome and reduce the number of disappointments. As mentioned earlier, there are already some suggestions for which behavioural traits will affect the strength of the relationship with the cat.[17]

Human–Cat Interactions

One of the main goals of our research group has been to establish a measure for relationship quality which equally considers both human and animal partners. During the course of this search, a number of interesting findings about the human–cat relationship in general have been made.[17,18,20]

It is possible to define an 'intention' to interact with a social partner by approach and/or vocal behaviour and to determine whether that 'intent' was successful, i.e. actually followed by an interaction. In one study an analysis was made of the proportion of interaction attempts by the owner or cat that were successful (i.e. the cat showed X 'intents' to interact and was successful in initiating an interaction in Y% of the cases). These data were then correlated with the total interaction time in the relationship. There was a significant **negative** correlation for the human data.[18] The more 'successful' the person was in initiating interactions with the cat, the **shorter** the total interaction time

in the relationship. Interpretation of these data are difficult, but it is possible that humans are capable of 'forcing' interactional wishes on the cat (e.g. approaching and stroking the animal), resulting in a 'success', but one that is only superficial. This suggestion was supported by a further result. When the proportion of successful intents to interact that were due to the cat was examined, this was found to be positively associated with total interaction time over all human–cat relationships. In other words, it is really the cat who decides how much interaction takes place, even though we are often given the impression that we are in control of the situation. Interestingly, the proportion of successful intents to interact that were due to the cat was lower in households with single owners, or single cats, but higher in cats living only indoors.[18] For persons living alone the cat becomes a 'significant other' and the owner is likely to initiate more interaction. In multiple-cat households, the animals are probably vying for the attention of their owners, who spend less time interacting with each of the cats than do the owners of single cats. Single cats may therefore need to initiate fewer interactions. In contrast, for indoor cats, the person becomes an important source of social contact and it is the cat who is likely to initiate more interactions.

It is possible to measure the degree to which the interactional 'goals' of each partner 'meshes' with those of the other[5] by measuring each partner's willingness to comply with, or fulfil the interaction wishes of its counterpart (shown by an 'intent' to interact). This measure for each partner in the human–cat relationship is significantly and positively correlated over all relationships studied. Thus, if the person complies with the interactional wishes of the cat, then at other times, the cat will comply with the interactional wishes of the person. The **more** willing the owner is to fulfil the cat's wishes, then the **more** willing the cat is to reciprocate.[18] This is a first indication that human–cat relationships are true social relationships, perhaps based on 'give and take' or even a rudimentary form of 'fairness'.

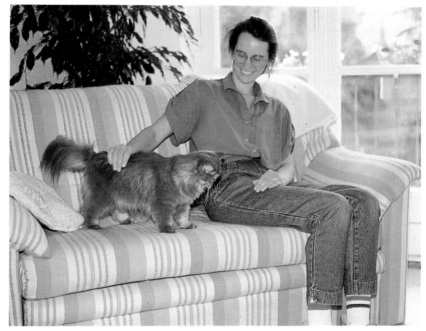

Fig. 7.4: Contact initiated by the cat led to longer interaction times.
© I.E.T./I.E.A.P.

Relationship Quality

Recent work has helped to explain both why human–cat relationships are so popular and how one might improve their quality.[17,18] The fact that the human–cat relationship can exist at low levels of willingness to comply with the partners' interactional wishes, as well as at high levels, allows a full range of different intensities of relationship from which people can choose and to which the cat adjusts. A symmetry exists in the relationships at all levels. An owner can increase or decrease his or her willingness to comply with the cat's interactional wishes. When one compares relationships showing high levels of compliance with those showing low levels of compliance, we find that high compliance on the part of the human is associated with acceptance of the cat's independence. This, in turn, is associated with a higher proportion of the intents to interact being due to the cat[18,21] and, therefore, a higher total interaction time. Thus, acceptance of a cat's independent nature is one of the secrets of a harmonious human–cat relationship.

Responsibilities of Cat Ownership

Cat owners need to fulfil more than just the cat's interactional wishes. When we accept a companion cat in our household, we are accepting responsibility to provide the animal with everything it needs, from social partners, to enough space, food and water. This is especially true for indoor cats, since cats allowed outside can often compensate for the mistakes we sometimes make inside the house. The importance of other cats as social partners, especially for indoor cats when the human partners are absent, has already been mentioned.[16,19,20] However, a general recommendation that a cat should always be kept with at least one other cat is incorrect. There are a number of cats which, because of poor early experiences or perhaps genetic make-up, are not sociable with other cats. Although these animals make good companions for humans, they should not be forced to live indoors with other cats.

The domestic cat, as a species, is quite flexible with respect to spatial requirements,[9] but

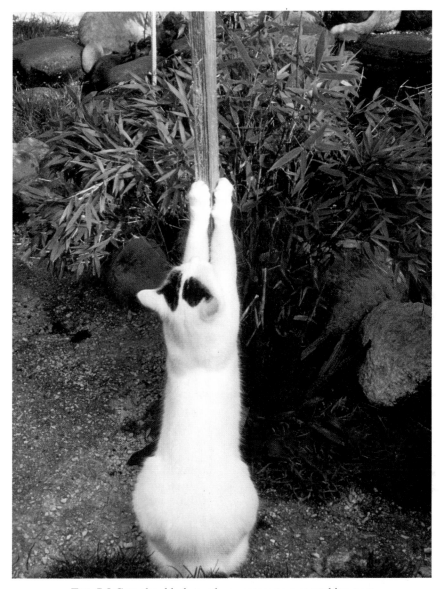

FIG. 7.5 Cats should always have access to a scratching post.
© I.E.T./I.E.A.P.

there is a limit to that adaptability. The smallest home ranges found in free-ranging cats are still larger than a one-room flat in the city! A fair proportion of cats showing behavioural disturbances come from small urban flats. However, the fact that not all indoor cats from small flats exhibit such problems indicates that it is possible to house these animals successfully, if the flat is properly 'furnished' and the owner is pre-pared to satisfy **all** of the cat's biological and psychological needs.

Experience at an animal behaviour clinic leads to the belief that the most important points and requirements to consider are:

- The proper number of social companions (ranging from no other cats up to one additional cat for each additional room in the flat).[20]

- Enough space that is structured so as to allow withdrawal into a quiet niche when contact with people or conspecifics is not desired.
- At least one litter tray per cat in the household, with the cats themselves deciding which one they utilise. These should not be placed alongside each other or beside food and should, of course, be cleaned regularly, always using the same brand of litter or making very gradual changes.
- A warm, dry and draught-free place to sleep, although a formal 'bed' is not required for a cat.
- Elevated look-out (and resting) posts. Cats prefer to rest at places where they have an 'overview' of what's going on.
- A scratching post, to allow proper care of the claws and, quite possibly, a demonstration of social status. Dominant cats tend to scratch before subordinate cats.[21]
- Stimulation, in particular, to release pent-up hunting motivation[25] and to reduce boredom (often achieved through play with objects).
- Well-balanced food (based on the nutritional requirements of cats and not people!) and water.
- Cat grass, especially for indoor cats, which may be a mechanical aid to digestion.

Living together with other cats (whether in the same household or outdoors) poses new problems for cats that originally evolved as territorial, solitary animals. Although they are quite capable of adjusting their social organisation system to a wide variety of ecological conditions,[8,9] dependent on the type of socialisation process they have gone through,[7] their reproductive and immune systems are still those of a solitary species and this requires compensation by humans, who are responsible for the socio-spatial organization of cats today. Therefore, neutering cats allowed outdoor access and immunisation against the most frequent cat illnesses is called for and ethically justifiable.[12,16,20]

In summary, recent scientific studies of the cat–human relationship has provided an interesting view of the extensive range of relationships which can exist between man and cat. This research has also given indications for how best to house cats to maximise their welfare, although in many cases cats seem to be less concerned about their owners and their housing conditions than the owners are about their cats.[18] The popularity of cats is increasing in many countries, no doubt due in part to their adaptability, but we must remain aware of the cat's needs in order to maintain a harmonious relationship. Future research on the behavioural needs of cats and their interactions with man should help us maximise the pleasure and benefits that we receive from our interactions with these intriguing animals.

References

1. Bergler, R. (1986) *Man and Dog: Psychology of a Relationship.* Blackwell Scientific Publications, Oxford.
2. Bergler, R. (1989) *Mensch und Katze. Kultur, Gefühl, Persönlichkeit.* Deutscher Instituts-Verlag, Köln.
3. Bradshaw, J. W. S. (1992) *The Behaviour of the Domestic Cat.* CAB International, Wallingford.
4. Fitzgerald, B. M. (1988) Diet of domestic cats and their impact on prey populations. In *The Domestic Cat: The Biology of its Behaviour.* Eds. D. Turner and P. Bateson. pp. 159–178. Cambridge University Press, Cambridge.
5. Hinde, R. A. (1976) On describing relationships. *Journal of Child Psychology and Psychiatry,* **17,** 1–19.
6. Hinde, R. A. and Stevenson-Hinde, J. (1976) Towards understanding relationships: dynamic stability. In *Growing Points in Ethology.* Eds. P. Bateson and R. A. Hinde. pp. 451–477. Cambridge University Press, Cambridge.
7. Karsh, E. B. and Turner, D. C. (1988) The human–cat relationship. In *The Domestic Cat: The Biology of its Behaviour.* Eds. D. C. Turner and P. Bateson. pp. 159–178. Cambridge University Press, Cambridge.
8. Kerby, B. and Macdonald, D. W. (1988) Cat society and the consequences of colony size. In *The Domestic Cat: The Biology of its Behaviour.* Eds. D. C.

Turner and P. Bateson. pp. 67–82. Cambridge University Press, Cambridge.

9. Liberg, O. and Sandell, M. (1988) Spatial organization and reproductive tactics in the domestic cat and other felids. In *The Domestic Cat: The Biology of its Behaviour*. Eds. D. C. Turner and P. Bateson. pp. 83–98. Cambridge University Press, Cambridge.

10. Meier, M. and Turner, D. C. (1985) Reactions of house cats during encounters with a strange person: evidence for two personality types. *Journal of the Delta Society*, **2**, 45–53.

11. Mertens, C. (1991) Human–cat interactions in the home setting. *Anthrozoös*, **4** (4), 214–231.

12. Mertens, C. and Schaer, R. (1988). Practical aspects of research on cats. In *The Domestic Cat: The Biology of its Behaviour*. Eds. D. C. Turner and P. Bateson. pp. 179–190. Cambridge University Press, Cambridge.

13. Mertens, C. and Turner, D. (1988) Experimental analysis of human–cat interactions during first encounters. *Anthrozoös*, **2** (2), 83–97.

14. Serpell, J. A. (1981) Childhood pets and their influence on adult's attitudes. *Psychology Reports*, **49**, 651–654.

15. Turner, D. C. (1988) Cat behaviour and the human/cat relationship. *Animalis Familiaris*, **3** (2), 16–21.

16. Turner, D. C. (1989) *Das sind Katzen. Informationen für eine verständnisvolle Partnerschaft*. Müller-Rüschlikon Verlag AG, Cham.

17. Turner, D. C. (1990) Owner assessment and the ethology of human–cat relationships. In *Pets, Benefits and Practice*. Ed. I. Burger. pp. 25–30. BVA Publications, London.

18. Turner, D. C. (1991) The ethology of the human–cat relationship. *Schweizer Archiv für Tierheilkunde*, **133**, 63–70.

19. Turner, D. C. (1991) Ethologie und die Mensch-Tier-Beziehung. In *Ethische Konflikte in der Tiernutzung*. Eds. H. Holzhey and A. Rust. pp. 32–40. Philosophisches Seminar der Universität Zürich, Zürich.

20. Turner, D. C. (1992). *Von Katzen und Menschen*. I.E.T., Hirzel and Zürcher Tierschutz, Switzerland.

21. Turner, D. C. (in press) *Mensch-Katze-Beziehung. Ethologische und Psychologische Aspekte*. Gustav Fischer Verlag, Jena.

22. Turner, D. C. and Bateson, P. (Eds.) (1988) *The Domestic Cat: The Biology of its Behaviour*. Cambridge University Press, Cambridge.

23. Turner, D. C. and Meister, O. (1988). Hunting behaviour of the domestic cat. In *The Domestic Cat: The Biology of its Behaviour*. Eds. D. C. Turner and P. Bateson. pp. 111–122. Cambridge University Press, Cambridge.

24. Turner, D. C. and Mertens, C. (1986). Home range size, overlap and exploitation in domestic farm cats (*Felis catus*). *Behaviour*, **99**, 22–45.

25. Turner, D. C., Feaver, J., Mendl, M. and Bateson, P. (1986). Variation in domestic cat behaviour towards humans: a paternal effect. *Animal Behaviour*, **34**, 1890–1892.

26. Widmer, F. and Turner, D. C. (1991). Katzen und Wasser. Ein erster Verhaltensvergleich zwischen Hauskatzen und Türkischen Van-Katzen. *Katzen Magazin*, **3**, 18–19.

CHAPTER 8

The Human–Dog Relationship

ANNE McBRIDE

Introduction

Much has been written about the human–dog relationship: its historical development,[21,22,25] the benefits of owning a companion dog[37] and the type of emotional bond which can be formed between owner and pet.[40] The human–dog relationship extends beyond the sphere of the companion animal as, throughout the world, dogs interact with people in a variety of other ways. They are used as assistance animals, for hunting, shepherding, tracking and rescue and as laboratory tools in medical and veterinary research. In all cases, a bond of some description is formed between man and dog, though little in the way of scientific study has been made of these relationships.[4,12]

In some instances, the emotional attachment formed may not be reciprocated as in the case of the dog who bonds strongly to a disinterested member of the family. Perhaps a more common example is that of people who, for religious or personal reasons, dislike dogs yet have to interact with them in public places. This chapter however, is concerned with the mutual relationships formed between owners and their companion dogs. Such bonds result from two-way interactions between man and dog. Both participants are linked,[15] their behaviour both modifying and being modified by that of the other.

In general, this reciprocity has not been given serious recognition either by scientists, veterinarians or the layman. Practically, this lack of attention has had important repercussions on the pet dog population. Whilst the majority of human–dog relationships are satisfactory and provide benefits to both participants, there is a proportion for whom this is not the case.[29] In the UK alone many thousands of dogs are destroyed because of behaviour problems. The more fortunate animals are given up for rehoming, though this in itself can lead to the exacerbation of the problems and the dog may be rehomed several times before it is finally settled, or euthanased.

The situation is gradually improving, as veterinarians and owners become increasingly aware that the risk of problems occurring can be reduced by appropriate socialisation and training. Likewise, there is growing awareness that problems, once they have developed, can frequently be resolved. The majority of these problems arise from dysfunctions in the human–dog relationship. They cannot be treated successfully unless a holistic approach is taken which includes the dynamics of the emotional attachments and communication signals used by both owner and dog. The basis of a successful relationship between man and dog (or any other species) is that the human knows the species, knows the breed and is able to communicate his intentions and wishes effectively.

Factors Affecting the Human–Dog Relationship

The Species

Whilst human–dog relationships are primarily concerned with social interactions, the responsible owner should be aware of the dog as a total organism. This includes awareness of the physical abilities and demands of the animal as well as an understanding of other areas of behaviour, such as reproduction, feeding and play.

The domestic dog's ancestral roots go back to the wolf. Whilst much work has been done on the social behaviour of the wolf, there has been less on that of the domestic dog. Until recently, it has been assumed that domestic dogs retain many of the communicative skills of the wolf and behaviourally resemble wolf pups. Indeed, much advice given in the treatment of behavioural problems is based on the premise that the dog is a neotenised wolf. Whilst this is a reasonable supposition and to date the best available, preliminary studies of breed differences in social communication suggest that the situation may not be quite that simple.

Introductory work by Bradshaw et al.[5] suggests that the more physically modified a breed is, the fewer elements of wolf-like behaviour it displays. Yet there does not seem to be a relationship between the degree of physical neotenisation and the retention of only infantile wolf behaviour. Of the breeds studied,[5] those showing the smallest repertoire of wolf-type signals (Norfolk Terriers, Shetland Sheepdogs and French Bulldogs) each showed one signal which is not seen in wolf cubs under 6 weeks of age, namely 'stand erect'. The finding that not all breeds produce the same signals as wolves, or even as each other, begs the further question of whether different breeds functionally employ these signals in different contexts. Much work needs to be done in this area. If different breeds do indeed 'speak different languages' then this could have interesting and far-reaching effects on various aspects of the human–dog relationship. However, given that this work is in its infancy, an understanding of wolf social behaviour and communication is the best available model for understanding our domestic dogs.[1,3,27]

Wolves are highly social animals which hunt and rear their young co-operatively. In order to maintain stability in their groups, they have evolved a hierarchical social system. This system functions to reduce intra-group aggression. Single-sex hierarchies are detectable in the wolf pack, with little cross-sex dominance. The hierarchies are pyramidal in structure with the most obvious rank differences between high-ranking individuals and less distinction between middle ranking adults and puppies. At the top of each hierarchy are the breeding, or alpha, male and female. These two have virtually exclusive breeding rights, suppressing breeding in the rest of the pack by antagonistic, but not usually aggressive, behaviour, although the alpha-female is often substantially more aggressive towards other females before and during the mating season.

Ritualised aggression, courtship, mating and parental behaviours serve to maintain the rank order with the minimum of physical harm being done to any party. Under natural conditions, where two animals, particularly males, are of too similar a status and antagonistic communication turns to aggression, then one would normally be ousted from the pack to live either as a solitary male or form a new pack. Often in the case of the domestic dog this is not an available option because the owner wishes to keep both dogs.

The stability of the hierarchy is dependent on individual animals using and responding to an extensive repertoire of communication signals. Communication is through the visual, tactile, olfactory and auditory sensory systems. A detailed discussion of canid communication is beyond the scope of this chapter, but has been extensively covered in other texts.[1,3,27] Aspects of human–dog communication will be discussed later in the chapter.

The Breeds

Though the dog is descended from the wolf, intensive selective breeding by man has produced over 400 separate breeds, many of which bear little physical resemblance to their forebears. It is important that the potential dog owner is aware of the breed attributes when initially selecting a breed. This may sound obvious, yet many pet owners are unaware of the associated traits of the breed they have chosen and problems can arise from not being aware of the psychological, as well as the physical requirements.

There have been several attempts to classify breeds of dogs by morphological features or by the function for which the animal was originally bred.[4] Such groupings include the gundogs, hounds, terriers, guard dogs, herding dogs and toy breeds. Whichever classification system is adopted, it does not alter an extremely important issue, namely, that breed characteristics have a profound influence on trainability and reactivity.[24,36] Often these are not taken into account when an individual purchases a puppy. An informal survey of owners attending puppy classes, asking 'What was your puppy bred for?' revealed a substantial degree of ignorance, with many owners stating that either they did not know or that the dog was bred for show. It should be realised that showing dogs at dog shows is not a function in its own right. Breeding dogs for show does **not** negate the basic behavioural traits of the breed. However, highly selective breeding for physical characteristics may distort the emotional traits of the breed, a situation currently under investigation in regard to a condition called 'rage syndrome' seen in some Cocker Spaniels in the UK.[32]

All groups of domestic dog have as their basic working characteristic a modification of the ancestral wolf-like predatory behaviour.[7,21] In dogs bred primarily for companionship, such as the Cavalier King Charles Spaniel,

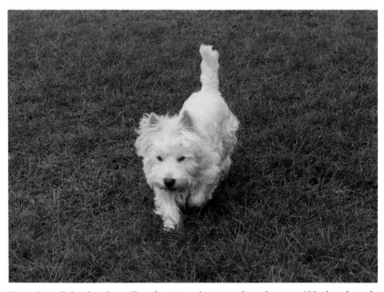

FIG. 8.1: Selective breeding by man has produced over 400 dog breeds, many of which bear little physical resemblance to their ancestor the wolf.

the predatory instinct has been drastically reduced by selective breeding, accompanied by a dramatic reduction in the size of the dentition. In contrast, in the herding dogs the hunting instinct has been inhibited at the point of the killing bite, whilst the stalk and herd elements of the predatory sequence have been emphasised. Similarly, the retrieving (bird-dog) breeds and the pointers have been bred for inhibited aggression.

In order for breeds, such as the retrieving and herding types, to perform successfully, they must be highly trainable. Part of their function is to respond to information from the human, such as indications of the direction in which to move. For other groups, the breed is expected to perform its function with little, if any, human guidance. In these breeds, traits of independent action have been emphasised and trainability has been of secondary importance. Consequently, these breeds are much more difficult to train. These include the terriers, in which the predatory instincts have been heightened so that these breeds are notoriously aggressive, often to other dogs or species which are far larger than themselves! Likewise, some of the guard breeds have been selected for heightened independent aggression. In those breeds whose original function was to act alone as guards, there was little requirement for them to be particularly trainable. Where a breed has a function which is merely an enhancement of a single behaviour, then low trainability is usually the outcome. The scent hounds are particularly good examples of this.

Low trainability is often confused with low intelligence as league tables published in the popular press testify. However, low trainability does **not** mean these dogs cannot respond to a positive programme of socialisation or to reward-based training methods. For example, terriers can have their aggression appropriately channelled to playing with objects and can even successfully undergo agility training. Low trainability merely indicates that these breeds tend to require more dedication on the part of the owner to motivate the dog to perform the commands requested.

Scott and Fuller[36] experimentally investigated emotional reactivity, trainability and problem-solving ability in breeds of the herding (Shetland Sheepdog), gun (Cocker Spaniel), scent hounds (Beagle), hunting (Basenji) and fighting (Fox Terrier) types. Tests for emotional reactivity included measuring heart rate under different circumstances, such as when the experimenter quietly entered or left the room, or when a mild electric shock was administered to the dog's leg. Trainability was tested with lead training and the dog's responsiveness to other simple commands. Investigation of problem-solving ability included maze and manipulation tests. No breed or group was consistently better than the others in all of the three investigative areas. Individual differences were also substantial. The overall conclusion of this work was that all breeds seem to be similar in terms of 'intelligence' but there are differences in which aspects of this 'pure intelligence' are most enhanced both within and, especially, between breeds.

More recently, Hart and Hart[24] investigated the characteristics of the 56 most popular breeds in the US. The investigation comprised a questionnaire survey of 96 veterinarians and dog obedience judges, who were asked to rank breeds on 13 different characteristics such as excitability, territorial defence, destructiveness and demand for affection. These were clustered into four traits; reactivity, aggression, trainability and investigation. Bradshaw[2] recently conducted a comparable study in the UK. Perhaps not surprisingly, differences were found between the two studies. For example, the Beagle, Irish Setter, Scottish Terrier, Standard Poodle and Airedale were considered less reactive and the Standard Dachshund, Dalmatian and Irish Setter less aggressive in the UK than in the US. These differences may be caused by several factors. For many breeds, particularly those of a foreign origin, there is a small genetic pool which means inbreeding can distort certain behavioural traits. Also, attitudes to dog management are different in the UK and the US. Many parts of the US have strict leash laws and dogs have little chance to socialise with their own kind. This may lead to a perception of increased aggression towards other dogs which is not necessarily a behavioural trait, but a consequence of insufficient socialisation. Likewise the tendency to restrict the dog's activity to the home may mean that breeds in the US are rated higher on territorial defence than they would be in the UK. Not all aspects of a dog's behaviour are related to breed traits. Another measure used by Hart and Hart was that of snapping at children. This trait is unlikely to be genetically influenced, other than as an indication of reactivity or aggressiveness. Such an indicator will therefore be misleading as the behaviour is influenced dramatically by an individual dog's experience, or lack of experience of children, another issue of socialisation.

While generalisations must be made with caution, as individual experience can greatly influence a dog's behaviour, owners should be aware of the original function of the breed and the behavioural traits which have been positively selected. Knowledge of the breed can greatly assist the owner in motivating the dog for training purposes and in preventing the development of behavioural problems, by being prepared for breed-specific behavioural tendencies such as digging, retrieving and swimming. A simple example will clarify this: companion animal behaviour counsellors see cases of aggression associated with possession of objects in Labrador Retrievers and Spaniels. In many instances this has developed because of misunderstanding and miscommunication between owner and dog. Gundogs have a basic behavioural trait to carry and retrieve objects and do not distinguish between their own toys and the owner's prize objects, such as shoes (a confusion further exacerbated if the owner gives the puppy an old shoe to play with!). Some owners, if unaware of this trait, respond in a confrontational manner to the puppy carrying what is perceived (by the owner) as an inappropriate object. From personal case histories, such confrontation can include hitting the dog, prizing its jaws open and even sprinkling pepper on its nose to make it sneeze and so release the object. The dog acts as if confused and fearful and, given sufficient experience of a confrontational reaction from its owner, will develop fear aggression when in possession of an object. Prevention of this situation is simple, but cure requires substantially more effort to rebuild trust on both sides of the canine–human partnership. Prevention merely requires that owners are made aware of the behavioural trait of retrieving. In the first few weeks of the puppy's being homed, owners should be encouraged to teach 'fetch' and 'drop', using positive reinforcement methods. Owners also need to realise their responsibility to remove valued objects out of the puppy's reach. Such preventative advice should be given by the breeder and be reaffirmed by veterinarian and trainer.

The above example illustrates an important point in the human–dog relationship. That is, the tendency of owners to attribute human thoughts and characteristics to their pets, in this instance attributing the ability to know right from wrong, of being able to understand the rationale behind the punishment (often inflicted after the puppy has chewed and discarded the object) and of being able to understand human attributions of assigning quality to objects. However, dogs do not think like humans and in order to enhance the dynamic relationship between pet and owner, it is necessary to understand means of communicating effectively with our canine companions.

Living in Harmony

Human–Dog Communication

Stability in canid social structures is dependent on effective communication which is equally important whether the animal is living in a conspecific group or with humans. Effective communication means that we should be able to make our dogs understand what is required from them in order that they may fit into our lifestyle. It also means that the dog is willing to comply with these requirements. In order for this to occur the

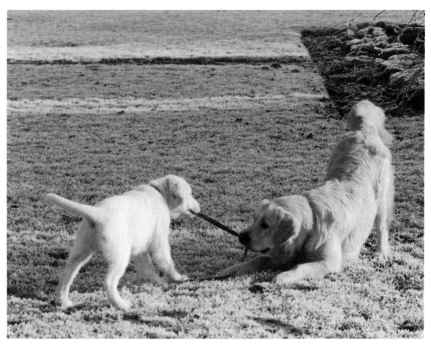

FIG. 8.2: An owner should be able to understand information being
conveyed by a dog through familiarity with the animal's body language.

dog must regard its owner as its leader. Leadership needs to be based on trust and on the dog's confidence in the reliability and constancy of the owner's behaviour. Effective communication has no requirement for physical strength, violence or confrontation. However, it does require that the owner be patient and be aware of the dog's limitations of understanding i.e. its cognitive abilities. The owner also needs to be familiar with the social behaviour of the domestic dog, of the specific traits of the breed and the individual dog's characteristics and learning history. An owner should be able to understand the information being conveyed by the dog through familiarity with the animal's body language and vocalisations. Whilst olfactory signals are of little use to the human communicator in dog–human interactions, there is some evidence that dogs not only recognise individual humans by their scent,[39] but also may detect different emotional states.[19]

In order to establish a positive relationship, it is necessary for the human to be aware of the signals he or she is using and how these may be translated by the dog, both in terms of the current interaction and in terms of the social situation as a whole. If, for instance, the human has acted consistently and persistently in ways which indicate their subordination and, subsequently, acts in a manner which is perceived as a status challenge by the dog, then an antagonistic response from the dog is likely. Unfortunately, through a lack of knowledge of canine social behaviour and communication, some owners find themselves in this type of situation and perceive the response from the dog as 'unprovoked aggression'. This aggression is not unprovoked, but stems from an underlying situation which has been created subtly and steadily by a series of *seemingly* unrelated incidents.

Many owners never have a problem with their dogs trying to assume higher status. This may be because their daily activities (e.g. not allowing dogs on to human beds) inadvertently but effectively communicate the owner's dominant position, or because the dog's temperament makes it readily subordinate to all humans. However, an awareness of the potential for a dog to seek leadership status is important for all owners.

A working knowledge of the social communication of the dog indicates several subtle ways in which the owner can communicate that they have a higher social status than the dog. These are described in depth in many popular dog behaviour books.[17,19] Owners can and should achieve authority over their dogs using methods which do not require strength or violence. Physically compulsive methods can merely serve to aggravate the situation, create distrust in the dog and lead to retaliation.

Non-compulsive methods require patience and consistency in order to achieve the required result. The prime consideration is that the authoritative figure (the human) has priority access to major resources. For example, food is a very important resource and in many societies, including that of the dog, the highest ranking individuals have precedence. Thus, the owner should feed the dog after having eaten, even if all the owner can manage is a token meal such as a cup of coffee. Owners should also have exclusive access to certain strategic areas of the environment such as beds and furniture. As in our own human society, increased height reinforces social rank, hence high-ranking individuals are often seated on a raised platform. Pack leaders are so called because they do indeed lead. Thus, another subtle cue to reinforce the human's authority is not to let the dog control the pace of the walk or pass through doorways before the person.

Another means of achieving authority is to teach the dog, from an early age, that the human has the right to handle it all over. Daily grooming sessions are invaluable for this, for both long- and short-haired animals. The dog can be accustomed to being touched all over by using rewards. For example, in order to earn a favourite titbit the dog should allow its paw to be briefly held. The principle of earning rewards is one which can be employed in a variety of situations in

order to achieve authority and will be discussed in more detail later in the chapter.

Games can have a different meaning to dogs. Games of 'rough and tumble', 'chase' and 'tug of war' can give the dog the impression that it is stronger or faster than the owner and should be avoided unless they can be controlled.[35] 'Throw–fetch' games and 'seeking object' games can provide a lot of fun whilst not involving any confusion of status. These status-maintaining procedures need to be sustained throughout the dog's life, otherwise the dog may perceive the owner to be relinquishing status and itself to be gaining increased status over the owner.

Owners need to be aware of the need for clarity and consistency in communication. Social signalling in the wolf and domestic dog entails very subtle visual cues, produced, for example, by ear and lip movements. Although we cannot produce the same types of movement, if we are consistent, dogs soon learn how to 'read' human body language, our non-verbal communication. As dogs are predators, they have a good ability to detect minute movements and thus are perhaps better at reading human movements than we are ourselves. We commonly hear of owners declaring that their dog 'knows exactly what I am thinking'. A more likely explanation is that the dog's perceptual and learning abilities has enabled it to understand the meaning of very slight body movements.[31]

Learning

Mammals begin to learn about their environment from the moment they are born. Indeed, there is some evidence that this process may begin whilst the foetus is in the uterus.[9–11] Though learning continues throughout life,[23] the young animal is more receptive to the acquisition of new information. There is a long-cherished myth amongst some people in the dog fraternity that training cannot begin until the dog is 6 months old. This is a fallacy which, thankfully, is fast losing credibility, since by this age, juvenile dogs have learnt much and often have developed 'problems' of lead pulling and jumping up. Learning is made far more difficult for both owner and dog, as the latter has to be **retrained** rather than trained!

In the first few weeks of life, much of what the puppy learns is through a process called **classical conditioning**. This is where an animal forms an association between an external event and an involuntary reaction. Indeed, this is the basis of the process of socialisation through which the puppy learns that the world is either a pleasant or a fearful place. Classical conditioning procedures can be used to great advantage, for example, associating visits to the veterinarian with special food treats, or associating the puppy's first experience of thunder with a distracting game. Classical conditioning can also produce unexpected negative results. For example, the puppy who is 'disciplined' by being swatted with a rolled-up newspaper may learn to associate newspapers with fear and thus, later, attack people carrying rolled-up newspapers. This example serves to reiterate the importance of realising that canine cognition is relatively limited. While the dog makes a simple connection between fear and the newspaper, it is quite likely that it made no connection with discipline for the original misdemeanour, especially if the punishment occurred after the event. Punishment which occurs after the event is meaningless to dogs and other animals, as no explanation for the punishment can be communicated.

Like other social animals, dogs learn many of their life skills by observing other members of the group. These skills may be positive, such as learning to come when called by following another dog, or negative, such as learning a fearful or aggressive response from another animal. Dogs can also learn from the human members of the pack. For instance, if the owner gets terribly excited and rushes to answer the telephone when it rings, the puppy will soon learn that this is an appropriate response and the owner will be accompanied by a barking, excitable dog—a behaviour which can soon turn into a problem as the owner never has an uninterrupted telephone conversation.

Perhaps the most important means by which domestic dogs learn about their social and physical environment is through a process called **operant conditioning**. The principle underlying this type of learning is that an action on the part of the animal can result in positive or negative reinforcement. Positive reinforcers can be thought of as rewards and increase the frequency of the behaviour which produces them. Negative reinforcers are consequences to be avoided or escaped from. They may be associated with pain and decrease the frequency of the behaviour which produces them. Traditional training methods using choke chains, and the more modern equivalents of shock and spike collars, employ the principle of negative reinforcement. A dog will learn to perform a behaviour in order to avoid the pain, if the negative reinforcer is applied at the correct time. If the timing is incorrect the dog may become confused and, in some cases, an incorrectly applied negative reinforcer may increase the behaviour it was designed to reduce. It is a quirk of human nature that many owners of beloved dogs are willing to employ these methods, even though it was shown experimentally, several decades ago, that positive reinforcement is an equally powerful training tool.[16] In addition, positive reinforcement has the advantage of reinforcing the trusting bond between owner and animal.[26] Many enlightened owners are now actively seeking training advice based on principles of positive reinforcement and a new genre of dog training books has recently become available.[18,35]

Research has shown[34,38] that, for learning to occur effectively and without causing stress to the animal, there must be constancy between the signal and the expected outcome of the animal's response. If this association is unreliable then the animal will become stressed and will respond inappropriately, possibly by doing nothing or becoming aggressive. This is akin to the human state when one cannot make up one's mind about what to do as one is unsure of the outcome. If owners are unaware of this, they can induce a similar state in their dog, merely by using the 'come' command (the signal) sometimes for positive reinforcement with a food reward or praise and also when they punish the dog. The dog may become agitated at the command, not knowing whether it will be praised or punished if it responds to the signal and returns to the owner.

Training

Whilst the principles of operant conditioning are the basis of dog training, deliberate training is not required for learning to occur. For example, if the dog barks at the postman and the postman goes away, barking has been reinforced by the consequence of the immediate departure of the postman. Training is merely guided learning. We do not teach our dogs to sit, we teach them how to be guided into the sit position in response to a verbal or physical signal. In order to train this we use positive reinforcement or reward; we pay the dog. Humans too learn and work for reward, which may be praise from a friend or colleague, the satisfaction of accomplishing something or for more basic needs which in the modern world are usually represented by money.

The currency of reward which we can apply to our dogs basically encompasses anything our dogs want. Powerful rewards for these social animals include praise, touch and casual eye contact. Food is an extremely powerful positive reinforcer. If a lot of food is used in training, this should be taken out of the dog's daily diet, which will serve the dual purpose of preventing the dog becoming obese and making the food reward more attractive since the dog has not consumed a large meal. Access to toys, play sessions, having the lead put on or taken off, doors opened, balls thrown etc. are also all potential rewards. Different breeds and individuals will be more strongly motivated by different positive reinforcers. Individuals will also vary from time to time with regard to which specific reward they will find motivating. A recently fed dog may not find titbits motivating but may be motivated by a ball. The owner should discover which rewards stimu-

late their dog's attention and use these to teach commands and reinforce those already learned.

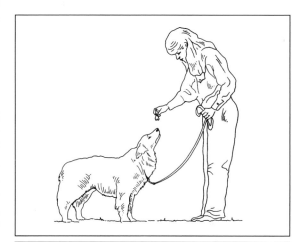

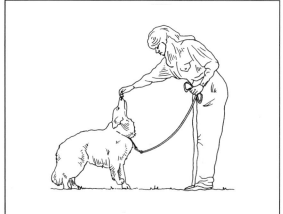

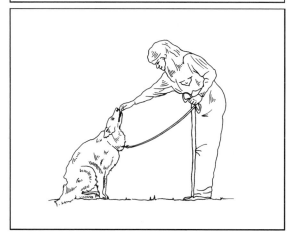

FIG. 8.3: The food reward method to guide a dog into a sit on command, demonstrating positive reinforcement.

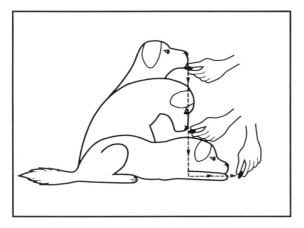

FIG. 8.4: Training the dog to respond to the 'down' command. The dog should be commanded to the sit position, then guided to 'down' by moving the food slowly along the floor, as indicated by the dotted line. The dog's head follows the food and the dog lies down.

If rewards are freely available then a dog is not going to bother to work for them. Most animals will take the easy route if it is presented to them. This often results in obedience only in specific situations, e.g. the dog who is only obedient in a training class or the obedience ring, but ignores the owner's command at other times. The probable cause of this difference is that, in the class or ring situation, the owner withholds all reward (praise, titbits, strokes, etc.) until the required response is forthcoming. In the home however, the dog may have free access to toys, is absentmindedly petted just for walking by or looking 'cute' or because it demands attention by gently pawing the owner. The dog has no need to work for praise and attention in this situation. Many people would also choose not to work if they were paid to do nothing! Making a dog earn rewards also helps to define the owner's place at the top of the dog's hierarchical social system. The member of a pack which has control of access to resources such as food, toys and attention is, by default, the higher ranking individual. In the dog–human pack this should be the human.

Not all owners wish to train their dogs to competition standards, a process requiring considerable time and dedication. However, the training of all dogs to a basic level of obedience is an important element of responsible dog ownership. Such basic training should include the dog walking quietly on the lead, coming when called, sitting on command and leaving objects (animate and inanimate) alone when so requested.

Punishment

Punishment occurs naturally in dog behaviour, for example, the older puppy that attempts to take its mother's food will be swiftly reprimanded with a low growl. Yet punishment in the dog or wolf pack is not common, nor is it related to issues such as barking or elimination. Punishment has little place in training and as already mentioned, physical punishment can result in later aggression either towards the owner or some other individual. If punishment is to be effective, it must occur whilst the behaviour is ongoing; hence punishment-based house training methods are not successful. Human parents have been successfully house training their own offspring using positive reinforcement for many generations. Applying the same principle to the dog, namely being aware of when the puppy needs to urinate or defecate, taking it to the appropriate place and rewarding it when it performs, is also extremely successful. For the dog owner, house training is helped by the puppy's instinct not to soil its bed area if it can help it, a claim which cannot be made for the human infant!

There is one form of punishment which can be useful and exploits the dog's social nature and need to be with its pack. This punishment involves simply ignoring the dog for a few minutes. Locking the dog outside for more than 2 or 3 minutes defeats the object of the exercise. Indeed, the dog need not be locked away. Totally ignoring unwanted behaviour, such as barking for attention, will reduce its frequency of occurrence. However, consistency is required, for if the dog sometimes receives a reward, the behaviour will be harder to remove. A regime of clearly and consistently ignoring (not rewarding) unwanted behaviour and rewarding wanted behaviour communicates the owner's wishes to the dog and thereby enhances the relationship.

Problem or Inappropriate Behaviour

Dogs, like other animals, attempt to behave in a manner which is, or appears to be, appropriate to the environment in which they find themselves. Indeed, from the dog's point of view, the **majority** of behaviours labelled as problematic are merely normal behaviours exhibited in response to a situation. Unfortunately, from the human viewpoint these behaviours are exhibited at inappropriate times or are deemed inappropriate in general. To refer back to an earlier example, the owner of the dog which displays his excitement by barking may not consider the dog to have a problem unless that barking disturbs his telephone conversations. The reality of the situation is that the dog does not have a behaviour problem, rather it is the owner who has a problem with the dog's behaviour. Another reported behaviour problem is the display of aggression by a dog towards its owner when the owner tries to make the dog do something. Again this is a perfectly normal response if the dog has been inadvertently taught that it is the leader of the human pack.

The factors underlying many problematic behaviours can be quite intricate and require advice from a professional behaviour counsellor, on referral from the animal's veterinary surgeon. Other problems can be resolved more easily, with recognition of the cause and solution arising from a consideration of the animal's social behaviour and learning capacity. Many problems can be prevented, or corrected with simple application of the principles of operant conditioning. Consider just two examples; jumping up and lead pulling. Puppies, like all dogs, have a behavioural need to investigate the scent of people they meet, hence their habit of sniffing

and of jumping up. If puppies are **consistently** only greeted when they are sitting and the human bends down to do so, then jumping up should never be a problem. This can be further extended so that the dog is only petted when sitting and only has his ball thrown when sitting, thereby setting standards for times when he meets strangers or comes across children playing ball.

Lead pulling can be prevented or corrected, but again patience and consistency are required. The reward the dog is seeking to obtain, by pulling on the lead, is to traverse from point A to B as fast as possible. Traditional methods of saying 'heel' and yanking on the lead are ineffective for the majority of owners. This is mostly down to the lack of an accurate sense of timing of when to inflict the negative reinforcement (i.e. yanking on the chain). The simpler, kinder way to train is based on positive reinforcement. The dog is **not** allowed the reward of moving forward, **unless** it is walking quietly by the owner. No command is even needed; it is enough that every time the dog pulls, the owner stops dead or changes direction. The golden rule is that if the dog pulls then neither dog nor owner moves in the desired direction. Such training takes time and owners should not try to teach walking to heel if they themselves are in a hurry. Attempting to rush training will invariably require a greater time input at some future stage when the dog has to beretrained.

In the same way that unwanted behaviours can easily be prevented, so they can inadvertently be encouraged. For example, saying 'get down' and pushing away the dog who jumps up actually provides the reward it was seeking, namely the owner's attention. It is better to stand still and totally ignore a dog which jumps up. Dogs soon learn what will earn them attention and it is not always what the owner would wish. Many owners rarely talk to or stroke a dog which is lying quietly. The owner tends to forget the dog when it is quietly behaving itself, so the dog learns that in order to get attention it needs to 'misbehave'. Gently stroking or talking to the dog who is lying quietly will serve to reinforce that behaviour.

It is important for owners to understand that dogs do not speak our language. Many owners unwittingly cause problems because they forget this simple fact. For example, young puppies can appear fearful of a new person; perhaps the puppy has previously only met women and is fearful of the first man it meets. The owner may try to reassure the dog by stroking it, talking to it and telling it that there is nothing to worry about. Unfortunately the owner may be reinforcing the dog's fearful behaviour for, from the dog's viewpoint, stroking and talking are positive reinforcers. Such misguided owner behaviour can result in a dog who has been trained to be fearful of men. It would be more productive to employ observational learning. If the owner approaches the stranger in a friendly manner, his or her behaviour will demonstrate the appropriate response and reassure the puppy that the stranger is not to be feared.

Responsibilities of Dog Ownership

A dog owner has many responsibilities both to the dog acquired and to their fellow citizens.

Responsibilities to the Dog

The quality of the dog's life is the total responsibility of the owner. There are many books available on dog care[13,14] and detailed discussion is beyond the scope of this chapter. However, there are a number of basic obligations which all owners should fulfil.

The dog is a social animal and the owner needs to spend several hours per day interacting with it. In addition, dogs need to be stimulated mentally, not only through training of basic commands but, also, through 'games' designed to employ their cognitive abilities.[35] Dogs need to be exercised every day. The demands for this will vary for each breed, but for many of the herding and hunting breeds this requirement can be considerable. Owners are also responsible for the physical health requirements of their dogs which include:

- correct feeding;
- regular and frequent grooming sessions, preferably daily for both short and long-coated breeds;
- weekly health checks when the owner can check for overgrown nails, cuts, lumps, ticks, fleas and sore eyes, ears and gums;
- regular worming—at least 6 monthly for adult dogs, or as recommended by the veterinary surgeon;
- annual vaccination, or as recommended by the veterinary surgeon.

Responsibilities to People

It is the owner's responsibility to ensure that their dog is well socialised (see *Chapter 6*), well trained and under control at all times. The law in many countries is extensive on this issue. For instance, in the UK owners are liable if their dog should cause a traffic accident and recent British legislation states that owners are liable for criminal prosecution and euthanasia of their dog should the dog injure or merely shock somebody.

Many areas now have anti-fouling laws to enforce what should be part of the basic responsibilities of the dog owner—namely the cleaning up of faeces deposited in public areas. Thus, owners should always carry a plastic bag or commercial scooping device for the collection and appropriate disposal of their dog's waste.

Finally, it is the owner's responsibility to consider the views of others. Not everyone holds positive attitudes to dogs. Some people are fearful of dogs, others may have negative views based on religious beliefs. In an ever more cosmopolitan world these attitudes should be respected. Consequently, the owner should have sufficient control over the dog in public places so that it does not interfere with an individual's personal space unless invited to do so. If a potential owner is not prepared to take on the responsibilities outlined above, then they should accept that they are not suitable as dog owners, whatever emotional fulfilment they may expect or desire, albeit unconsciously, from the relationship.[28,40]

The human–dog relationship has existed for many generations and is likely to continue for many more. Recently it has undergone substantial change with the increased interest in show breeds and in ownership for purely companionship purposes. In addition, the increase in pet ownership in our towns and cities means that dogs are having to interact with many unfamiliar humans and conspecifics during the course of their lives. In order for the dog–human relationship to succeed in its new role, it is important that both owners and non-owners have an understanding of dog behaviour. It is also the responsibility of the breeder, veterinarian and, most of all, the owner to ensure that his or her dog has had every opportunity to develop into an emotionally stable, controllable individual.

Dog ownership, like the rearing of children, requires dedication, understanding, time and effort, and the responsibilities last a lifetime. It should not be undertaken lightly and, to be truly successful, it should be well prepared for. Potential owners should research thoroughly those breeds in which they are interested, in order to ensure that the physical and mental requirements of the breed can be fully met. Once the dog is obtained, if not before, the breeder and veterinarian have a responsibility to direct the owner towards information concerning dog behaviour, development, positive training methods[33] and where local recommended socialisation and training classes can be found. The pet owner is becoming a more informed, discerning individual and it is to the professionals' long term advantage that they are able to recommend training classes rather than simply allow advertising in their waiting rooms. Finally, the owner needs to be aware of how to become and remain the dog's respected, loved and trusted pack leader,[17,19] in order to maximise the pleasure and benefits that they receive from dog ownership.

References

1. Abrantes, R. A. B. (1987) The expression of emotions in man and canid. In *Canine Development throughout Life*. Ed. A. T. B. Edney. Waltham Symposium No. 8. *Journal of Small Animal Practice*, **28**, 1030–1036.
2. Bradshaw, J. W. S. (1994) Personal communication.
3. Bradshaw, J. W. S. and Nott, H. M. R. (in press) Social and communication behaviour of companion dogs. In *The Domestic Dog: its Evolution, Behaviour and Interactions with People*. Ed. J. A. Serpell. Cambridge University Press.
4. Bradshaw, J. W. S. and Wickens, S. M. (1992) Social behaviour of the domestic dog. *Tijdschrift voor Diergeneeskunde*, **117**, 50S.
5. Bradshaw, J. W. S., Wickens, S. M. and Goodwin, D. (1994) Dogs and wolves: Do they really speak the same language? *Association of Pet Behaviour Counsellors' Newsletter*.
6. Bradshaw, J. W. S., Goodwin, D., Lea, M. and Whitehead, S. L. (1995) Behavioural characteristics of pure bred dogs in Britain. *Veterinary Record* (in press).
7. Coppinger, R., Glendinning, J., Torop, E., Mathay, C., Sutherland, M. and Smith, C. (1987) Degree of behavioural neoteny differentiates canid polymorphs. *Ethology*, **75**, 89–108.
8. Doty, R. L. and Dunbar, I. F. (1974) Attraction of beagles to conspecific urine, vaginal and anal sac secretion odours. *Physiology and Behaviour*, **12**, 325–333
9. De Casper, A. and Fifer, W. (1980) Of human bonding: newborns prefer their mothers voices. *Science*, **208**, 1174–1176.
10. De Casper, A. J. and Sigapoos, A. D. (1983) The intrauterine heartbeat: a potent reinforcer for newborns. *Infant Behaviour and Development*, **6**, 19–25.
11. De Casper, A. J. and Spence, M. J. (1986) Prenatal maternal speech influences newborn's perceptions of speech sounds. *Infant Behaviour and Development*, **9**, 133–150.
12. Estep, D. Q. and Hetts, S. (1992) Interactions, relationships and bonds: the conceptual basis for scientist–animal relations. In *The Inevitable Bond*. Eds. H. Davis and D. Balfour. pp. 6–26. Cambridge University Press.
13. Evans, J. M. and White, K. (1988) *The Book of the Bitch*. Henston.
14. Evans, J. M. and White, K. (1988) *The Doglopaedia*. 3rd edn. Henston.
15. Fentress, J. (1992) The covalent animal: on bonds and their boundaries in behavioural research. In *The Inevitable Bond*. Eds. H. Davis and D. Balfour. pp. 44–71. Cambridge University Press.

16. Ferster, C. B. and Skinner, B. F. (1957) *Schedules of Reinforcement.* Appleton-Century-Crofts, New York.

17. Fisher, J. (1991) *Why Does My Dog?* Souvenir Press.

18. Fisher, J. (1992) *Dogwise; The Natural Way to Train Your Dog.* Souvenir Press.

19. Fogle, B. (1990) *The Dog's Mind.* Pelham Books.

20. Fox, M. W. (1975) *Understanding Your Dog.* Book Club Associates, London.

21. Fox, M. W. (1978) *The Dog: Its Domestication and Behaviour.* Garland STPM Press, New York.

22. Fox, M. W. (1978) Man, wolf and dog. In *Wolf and Man, Evolution in Parallel.* Eds. R. L. Hall and H. S. Sharp. Academic Press.

23. Gross, R. D. (1992) *Psychology, The Science of Mind and Behaviour.* Hodder and Stoughton.

24. Hart, B. L. and Hart, L. A. (1988) *The Perfect Puppy.* W. H. Freeman and Co.

25. Howey, M. O. (1975) *The Cults of the Dog.* C.W. Daniel Limited.

26. Kosarczyk, E. (1993) The use of dog–human interaction as a reward in instrumental conditioning and its impact on dogs' cardiac regulation. In *The Inevitable Bond.* Eds. H. Davis and D. Balfour. pp. 109–131. Cambridge University Press.

27. Nott, H. M. R. (1992) Social behaviour of the dog. In *The Waltham Book of Dog and Cat Behaviour.* Ed. C. Thorne. pp. 97–114. Pergamon Press, Oxford.

28. O'Farrell, V. (1994) *Dog's Best Friend; How Not to be a Problem Owner.* Methuen.

29. Patronek, G. J. and Glickman, L. T. (1994) Development of a model for estimating the size and dynamics of the pet dog population. *Anthrozoös,* **VII,** 25–41.

30. Peters, R. P. and Mech, L. D. (1975) Scent marking in wolves. *American Scientist,* **63,** 628–637

31. Pfungst, O. (1965) *Clever Hans (the Horse of Mr von Osten).* Ed. R. Rosenthal. Holt, Rinehart and Winston, New York.

32. Podberscek, A. (1994) Rage syndrome — facts, fiction and current investigations. *Recent Advances in Pet Behaviour Therapy.* Transcript of Waltham APBC Symposium,

33. Pryor, K. (1991) *Don't Shoot the Dog.* Bantam New Age Books.

34. Rescorla, R. A. (1968) Probability of shock in the presence and absence of CS in fear conditioning. *Journal of Comparative and Physiological Psychology,* **66,** 1–5.

35. Rogerson, J. (1992) *Training your Dog.* Popular Dogs.

36. Scott, J. P. and Fuller, J. L. (1965) *Genetics and the Social Behaviour of the Dog.* University of Chicago Press, Chicago.

37. Serpell, J. A. (1986) *In the Company of Animals: A study of Human–Animal Relationships.* Basil Blackwell, Oxford.

38. Seligman, M. E. P. (1971) Phobias and preparedness. *Behaviour Therapy,* **2,** 307–320.

39. Settle, R. H., Somerville, B. A., McCormick, J. and Broom, D. (1994) Human scent matching using specially trained dogs. *Animal Behaviour,* **48,** 1443–1448.

40. Veevers, J. E. (1985) Social meaning of pets: Alternative roles for companion animals. In *Pets and the Family,* Ed. M. B. Sussman. pp. 11–30. Haworth Press.

CHAPTER 9

Relationships with Other Pets

IAN ROBINSON and ANNE McBRIDE

Introduction

The term **companion animal** is often interpreted as being synonymous with dog or cat. These are the species most often seen, as they are visible outside the owner's home and are the only domesticated animals which retain an association with man without being caged, tethered or otherwise restrained. Yet, the most common pets or companion animals are probably fish. Humans keep a wide variety of species, both vertebrate and invertebrate, as pets. The more familiar species, such as rabbits, budgerigars, hamsters, cold water and tropical fish, can be found in many pet shops. More unusual species include snakes and other reptiles, exotic mammals and birds, as well as invertebrates such as tropical spiders, giant land snails and stick insects.[26] A recent survey of UK magazine circulation figures[13] illustrates both the variety and popularity of these 'alternative' companion animal species.

Horses, although often kept for sporting or competitive purposes, may also be considered as companion animals. Although for centuries the horse was the principal means of transport, its population declined as farm work and transport became increasingly mechanised. In the last 40 years, however, there has been an increasing interest in riding as a sport or hobby and in some developed countries the horse population is possibly greater now than it has ever been.

This chapter will examine human interactions with pets other than cats and dogs and will consider some of the responsibilities of ownership. Owing to the wide variety of species kept as companions and the consequent variety of needs, only a brief introduction can be given. However, specialist books are available for potential owners who require further information.

Man's Association with the Horse

Historical Associations

The horse was a major factor in the development of many human cultures, although the history of its domestication is unclear. Initially, horses were hunted as a source of food, as depicted in 15,000-year-old cave paintings found in France and Spain.[9] There is also some evidence that they may have been kept captive from around 14–15 thousand years ago. Images of horse heads from this era contain lines which resemble a halter[25] although this may have been an attempt to depict muscle lines on the head. There are some suggestions that horses may have been kept captive even earlier. Some 30,000-year-old horse teeth have been found which show a similar sort of wear to that produced by modern horses during crib biting. Since biting on hard objects is unknown in wild equids and only occurs in horses which are regularly tethered or stabled for long periods of time, this suggests that the horse was confined by man, although not necessarily domesticated.[25]

The first evidence for horses being ridden comes from an analysis of 6000-year-old horse teeth found in the Ukraine[1] which showed dental wear of the type normally caused by a bit. Horses fitted with bits could have been ridden or driven, but there is evidence that horses were also kept in corralled herds at this time.[1] As these horses could not have been moved in any numbers without mounted herdsmen, it is likely that at least some horses were ridden. No tooth wear attributable to a bit has been found in horse remains older than 6000 years and no equivalent wear has been found in modern feral horses which have not been ridden.[1]

Other archaeological evidence suggests that from about 5000 years ago there was an increasing tendency to use horses and asses for work. South-west Asian art from around 5000 years ago shows horses being ridden and as pack animals.[44] Selective breeding with the natural size variation found in horses from different areas gradually modified the horse into light and heavy varieties.[44] However, there is considerable debate regarding the genetic origins of modern horses and ponies. Such discussion is beyond the scope of this chapter, but reviews can be found in other texts.[9,30,34]

The impact that horse riding would have made on human societies has been estimated by examining the impact of the horse in the New World in the late 17th century. In North America, there is evidence that the horse had reached the Plains Indians before guns and European traders.[25] The horse gave

Plains Indians the ability to travel 2–3 times further and faster than they could on foot. This caused an increase in warfare as traditional ethnic boundaries, which previously had been based upon pedestrian travel distances, were contested. The horse was also an easily stolen standard of wealth. On the positive side, the horse stimulated greater trade by providing increased mobility and a means of transporting goods more efficiently.

Throughout history, the lifestyles of certain human groups became closely integrated with the horse. For example, the Russian Cossacks, the Argentinean gauchos, the North American Plains Indians and the American cowboys were all 'horsemen' and developed a reputation for being fearless, aggressive, proud and defiant. Association with the horse seemed to give a heightened sense of self worth in both a literal and symbolic sense and riding still seems to provide a symbolic image which makes a horse desirable over and above its use as transport. Lawrence[25] reports that if transportation had been the main issue, then several African populations would have ridden the quagga rather than the horse. Until the mid-19th century the quagga was a common equid in central and southern Africa. It was docile, easily tamed and trained and adapted for the local environment. However, quaggas were hunted to extinction by English and Boer farmers who considered them to be vermin. Horses were imported for riding at great expense because of the belief that only a true horse represented status and was therefore the only animal suitable for a colonist.

Horses in Society

There has been less research on understanding the human–horse relationship than with dogs or cats, although the types of human–horse interactions may be more varied and complex. Humans can interact with a horse in many different ways; from those who have occasional rides at weekends or during holidays, to those who keep the same animal for 30 years. Other people with a sporting interest may keep a number of horses and have a turn-over of individual animals as they strive for increased performance at a sport. There are also groups who use horses as part of their work (e.g. mounted police), or for whom the horse forms links with ancestral traditions and lifestyles (e.g. North American Plains Indians, gypsies). Such a wide range in type and intensity of interaction is likely to be reflected in a variety of human–horse relationships.

A study of the Crow Indians of Montana, a Northern Plains Indian tribe, showed how their entire society and culture changed after acquisition of the horse in the early 18th century.[24,25] The Crow held horses in high esteem; they represented prestige and wealth and became the main currency of exchange. When this tribe were defeated and confined to reservations in the late 19th century, loss of the horse contributed to the destruction of their culture. Today however, the Crow have regained the horse as part of their culture and horses are kept on Crow reservations. Competitions and other forms of recreation with horses have replaced traditional activities of hunting and war.[24,25]

The Crow's respectful relationship with horses is in contrast to aspects of modern day rodeo events in the US. Some events involve capturing, subduing, saddling and then riding a wild horse, a symbolic re-enactment of the taming of the West, emphasising man's control over nature. Along similar lines other rodeo events show man and horse working in harmony to subdue and control cattle. The American cowboy is often used to portray a lifestyle of rugged freedom, in contrast to the more aristocratic associations seen with horses in Europe, yet even the cowboy developed an elitist view and considered himself superior to the non-mounted farm worker.[23,24]

A study of the American mounted police[24] showed that police horses were perceived as a great asset since they accentuated police presence, gave the police increased visibility and the presence of mounted police officers appeared to reduce street crime. Police horses have also been reported to reduce public hostility towards and facilitate conversation with police officers. This socialising effect is similar to that reported for other species.[17,31,33] The general rule for mounted police is that one officer works with only one horse. They spend a lot of time with their horses each day and develop a sense of trust with the animal enabling them to predict how it will react to most situations. Officers report a close relationship with their horses and they often feel great resentment if they are forced to lend their horse to another person.

Many studies of people living and working with horses have shown how riding elevates the status of the rider both literally and symbolically, giving increased power and an increased sense of power. This perhaps explains why, historically, riding was reserved for the ruling elite. Today, although the availability of land and the high cost and time involvement in horse care may reduce the possibility of ownership for many people, the availability of riding establishments means that riding and interactions with horses are no longer restricted to the upper classes. Despite this, some studies[25] suggest that people who ride or handle horses seem to receive an elevation of status within their own social order. In many parts of Europe this elevated status may come from historical associations between horses and the landed gentry. In the US, riding is associated more with the tradition of the Old West, as represented by the cowboy,[2] and with a life of freedom. Some equestrian activities such as fox hunting still perpetuate traditional aristocratic associations and in sporting events such as dressage, there remains strict adherence to prescribed behaviour, clothing and styles of riding. The exact reasons for elevated status from associations with a horse are likely to be influenced by many factors. It has however been turned to beneficial effect in the use of horses as therapy for disabled people (see *Chapter 5*). Whilst associations with horses may elevate an individual's status within a social group, there are occasions where close association with the horse has caused rejection by other groups. When the

Tartars and the gypsies appeared in medi-aeval Western Europe, they were rejected and stigmatised because they were considered to have an unnatural closeness to horses.[10]

The Human–Horse Relationship

Most privately owned horses differ from other companion animals in that they are bought for a purpose, to be ridden, rather than as companions. A second major difference between horses and other pets is that whereas most pets are ideally kept by one family for their entire lives, horses usually have several owners and may be specifically bought as a temporary mount. This is especially true for horses or ponies bought for children because of the need to match the size and ability of the child to the animal. Thus, as a person ages or their riding ability improves, they may own a number of different animals. This change in ownership may alter the relationship with a horse. Jones[18] reports that many owners felt closer to their first animal than they did to those they owned subsequently.

In contrast to the detailed investigations made of human relationships with dogs and cats[2,3] (see *Chapters 7 and 8*), little work has been conducted with horse owners. In one study, 25 male and 25 female horse owners in the USA, were asked to indicate words and phrases from a checklist of 300 items, which corresponded to themselves.[21] The horse owners were found to show high levels of assertiveness and self-concern, but low levels of cooperativeness, novelty-seeking and nurturance. More specifically, male owners tended to be more aggressive and dominant, but showed lower levels of expressiveness, that is they corresponded to the traditional Western cowboy stereotype. Female owners tended to be more easy going and low in aggressiveness, again corresponding to traditional female sexual stereotypes.

Brown[7] observed 40 adult and 40 child horse owners who were exhibiting their animals at a show and compared their behaviour with a similar group of people exhibiting at dog shows. She found that female horse owners were more affectionate and interactive with their animals than males, who tended to be more punitive and

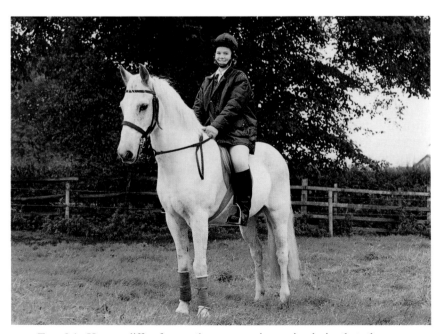

Fig. 9.1: Horses differ from other companion animals in that they are normally bought for a purpose other than companionship.

instrumental. This is in contrast to the dog owners where women tended to issue commands to their dogs, whereas men were more likely to solicit attention from their dogs. There was, however, a wide degree of variation within each sex. In a second study, Brown[7] studied 39 female and 20 male horse owners and 40 female and 39 male dog owners outside the show environment. Each subject's personality was assessed using a number of questionnaires. Male horse owners were found to be more dominant than females and in contrast to the study at dog shows, male dog owners were also more dominant than females. However, female horse owners and male dog owners showed similar levels of dominance. From these results Brown suggests that because of their size and power, horses are perceived as a greater dominance threat and so men interact in a more dominant and punitive manner relative to their interactions with dogs. The suggestion that female owners were more affectionate than males was supported by interviews with children[18] where both boys and girls gave the impression that boys cared less about their animals than did girls.

From interviews conducted with horse owners and riders, Jones[18] reported differences between types of riders which she divided into three broad groups. Members of the first group were termed **achievers** as they were mainly concerned with becoming accomplished riders. The second group were more concerned with the personal relationship with their horses and were termed **relators**. The third group were more interested in riding as a sport and this attitude was more prevalent amongst boys. Jones argued that although the achievers valued the utility of their horses, this did not mean that they did not love their animals. The time spent training together may create a closer relationship than that experienced by relators. Jones also reports an uneven sex ratio among young riders and notes that a number of children were teased at school about their horse ownership. There was a feeling that children considered riding to be a 'girls' sport'. As boys are much less likely to engage in cross-sex activities than girls, there is likely to be more pressure on boys to conform and thus not to ride.[18]

These studies give an indication of the

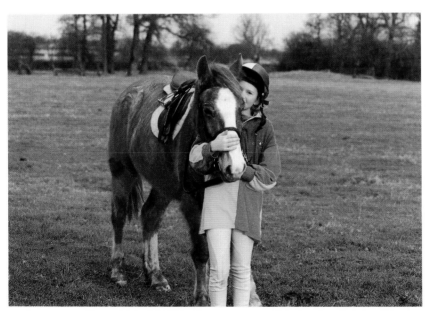

FIG. 9.2: Studies have suggested that female horse owners are more affectionate toward their horses than are male owners.

personality types of some horse owners. However, it is not possible to determine whether ownership and riding of horses promotes greater displays of characteristics such as dominance, or whether people with those character traits are more likely to become horse owners because it allows them to demonstrate these traits. To date, studies have only been conducted on small samples of owners. As indicated earlier, many people from a variety of backgrounds own or ride horses. Further research across a wider variety of owners and riders in a number of countries is required to obtain a clearer understanding of the human–horse relationship.

Responsibilities of Horse Ownership

A greater number of people ride rather than own horses. These people can receive great benefits and enjoyment from such associations without needing to know anything about horse feeding or care. This is perhaps equivalent to our association with the car where it is possible to drive throughout one's adult life without fully understanding how the car works. For horse owners, however, a great deal of time and energy is spent on care. Many books have been written on the subject of horse care and nutrition[5,14,27,41] and, in contrast to cats and dogs, training courses exist in some countries to educate owners on practical aspects of care and management. It is not possible to give a detailed discussion of horse care in this chapter, however, some elements of horse behaviour and their implications for horse welfare will be considered.

All equids are social mammals and in natural conditions tend to live in groups. For free-living domestic horses, the basic social organisation consists of a permanent group of a stallion with a harem of a few females. Each group has a home range which overlaps with that of neighbouring groups and the size of the home range varies depending on food availability. Males who are unable to win a harem tend to live together in bachelor groups.[30] Studies of free-living domestic horses

have shown that this basic social system can vary in response to local conditions, with harems tending to be larger and ranges smaller if food is plentiful.[37] Studies of ponies in the New Forest, England,[37] have shown that when stallions are rare, social groups are formed without them during winter months. These groups tend to be small and based around the families of one or more mares. During the spring and summer these groups join together into temporary harems which may have a sex ratio of 1 male to 60 females. This sex ratio is artificially maintained by the removal of stallions from the forest.

All horse species forage mainly on fibrous foods which are digested in the hindgut.[41] The horse's digestive system is less efficient than that of ruminants and so they rely on processing large quantities of food. The digestive process is also able to cope with poor quality foods so that horses are able to live in habitats which would be unsuitable for ruminants. The need for a large intake of food means that horses spend around 60% of the day and night foraging and this can rise to 80% in poor habitats.[30] This lifestyle of free-living, social grouping and almost continuous foraging contrasts dramatically with that of many captive individuals. Horses are often stabled alone for large parts of the day and may receive a large proportion of their energy requirements in the form of concentrated and refined foods which can be eaten in a few minutes. These restrictions can sometimes lead to displays of inappropriate behaviour.

The occurrence of stereotypical behaviour in horses is well known and has been described by many authors.[6,15,16,20,44] Such behaviour can include wind-sucking (which involves swallowing or expelling air), crib biting (where the animal makes wind-sucking movements but either rests its upper incisors on some solid object, or grips an object such as the stable door between upper and lower incisors), head nodding, stall walking and weaving (where the horse makes repeated movements with no obvious function). Such behaviour rarely occurs in horses living in a complex environment which is appropriate to their needs. It is usually seen where there is confinement, some form of frustration, or where the environment is unpredictable. Social isolation increases the likelihood that this sort of behaviour will be shown.

Traditional methods of control attempt to prevent the stereotypy occurring by either removing objects, or by restricting movements.[20] However, these do not address the cause of the problem and are likely to generate additional frustration for the animal. It is becoming increasingly recognised that stereotypies are an animal's response to stress generated by some aspect of its living conditions. Thus, a more enlightened approach is to attempt to treat the cause of the problem by modifying the environment. In fact, it has been argued[6] that if a horse performing a stereotypy is not causing direct damage to itself, then it should be treated not by blocking the action but by addressing its housing and management.

Horse management should take the horse's needs into account but these must not be judged only from the human perspective. A stable may appear boring and monotonous to a human observer but may not cause problems for the horse if other needs, such as availability of forage and companions, are met. In contrast, if a horse is displaying stereotypic behaviour, this suggests that there is a problem with the environment, however suitable it may appear to the human eye.

Many aspects of horse care are based on convenience or traditional practice, rather than an understanding of the animal's needs. Increasingly, an enlightened approach to animal welfare is improving the living conditions for many species. As increased leisure time leads to the increased popularity of recreational riding, it is hoped that there will be a corresponding increase in understanding of the biological needs of horses.

Relationships with other Pets

Adults, as well as children, can form important relationships with pets other than dogs, cats and horses.[38,43] This is particularly true where the species is long-lived. Longevity fulfils one of the requirements for the formation of such relationships, namely prolonged physical contact.[22] Some of the more obvious species in this category are tortoises, parrots and even rabbits which can live for a decade or more. Less obvious perhaps are the relationships formed by owners with snakes, spiders and even slugs,[36] species which, whilst long-lived, are not perceived as being particularly social or interactive. Relationships are also facilitated by similarities in the social and communication systems of the interacting species. There are large differences in the methods of communication used by many of these species compared to those of man. Thus, it is likely that relationships formed with small mammals, reptiles and invertebrates are primarily one-way, that is the non-human participant interacts but does not form a relationship. However, given that these animals are so popular, the owners must be deriving some sort of satisfaction from the relationship. This may involve the owner's desire to nurture living things or the owner may simply derive pleasure from observing animals. For instance, following the acquisition of goldfish by non-institutionalised elderly people, comments indicated that the owners had formed a relationship with the fish. These included statements such as 'they depend on me to feed them' or 'their antics make me laugh'.[38]

It is part of modern western folklore that pets are good for children, giving them a sense of responsibility, as well as perhaps initiating them into the mysteries of birth and death. The smaller species are often considered primarily as 'children's pets' and certainly strong bonds can be formed with such pets in addition to those formed with the family dog or cat. Strong bonds formed in childhood with a special pet can affect attitudes towards nature, the environment and humanity in later life.[35] The 'special importance' of the pet may reflect the child's exclusive ownership of and right of access to it, as compared to the shared ownership and shared access to the family cat or dog. Another important aspect is the physical

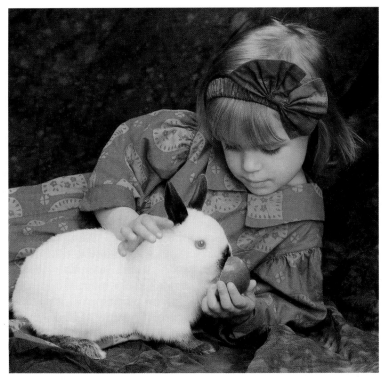

FIG. 9.3: Strong bonds formed in childhood with a special pet can affect
attitudes towards nature, the environment and humanity in later life.

manageability of many, so-called, 'children's pets'. Hamsters and rabbits tend to be small and can be easily handled by a young child.

In addition to the large numbers of shows held for dogs and cats, many other species have clubs and competitive shows. These provide a considerable amount of social interaction, which can become all-encompassing for those whose business endeavours, such as commercial breeding, means that their friendship networks and business contacts become merged. In this world the animal serves a function similar to that of a vintage car to car buffs or stamps to philatelists. There may be little, if any, bonding on the part of the human. Although bonds may be formed with a few individual animals, the high turn-over of animals between different owners and the disposal of stock 'unsuitable for show' to the pet market suggests that such bonding is uncommon especially with the larger breeders, where

exhibition is the chief reason for keeping the animals.[28]

A study by Kidd *et al.*[21] suggested that tortoise and turtle owners were hard-working, reliable and upwardly mobile, whereas bird owners were outgoing and expressive, with female bird owners showing high levels of dominance. However this study has only touched the surface of what must be a complex and varied range of human–animal interactions and relationships.

The remainder of this chapter will consider interactions with humans from the animal's viewpoint and its implications for the welfare of the pet.

Responsibilities of Ownership

Cats, dogs, snakes, other reptiles and spiders can be considered to be primarily predatory species. In contrast, the small mammal

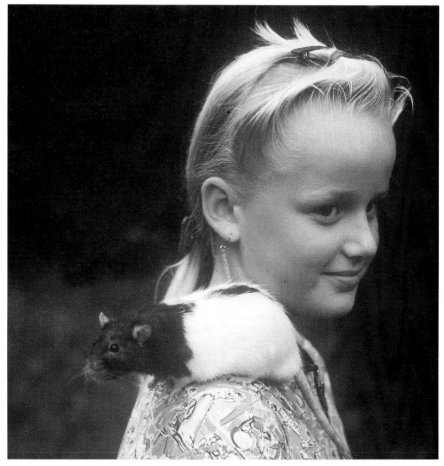

FIG. 9.4: Gentle handling of smaller pets when they are young can habituate
them to close contact with humans.

species commonly kept as pets, namely the rodents and lagomorphs (rabbits), are basically prey species. For such animals vigilance and evasion of potential predators are a constant condition pervading their daily life and activities, though this might not always be obvious to the human observer. It therefore follows that many of these animals will not naturally perceive humans as benign aspects of their environment.[8]

There are some behaviour patterns which we immediately recognise as anti-predator tactics: the rabbit which kicks when handled, or the hamster which bites. However, there may be more subtle changes in behaviour such as increased vigilance or a reduction in time spent feeding or grooming. These can be considered as welfare issues, especially as they may have long term consequences for the animal's health. For example, the pet rat, hamster or mouse kept in a cage which is located in a noisy, well-lit part of the house could suffer long term detrimental consequences,[19] since these species are primarily nocturnal. The responsible owner needs to be aware of the animal's natural daily rhythm and attempt to strike a balance between interacting with the animal and allowing time for it to rest and feed in an undisturbed location.

Other aspects of the environment also need to be considered. Most animals and certainly the small mammals we keep as pets can hear far higher-pitched sounds than we can. This is also true for fish which 'hear' by sensing tiny changes in the movement of the water. Thus, locating a cage, or fish tank, near household equipment which emits substantial levels of ultrasound can mean the animal is constantly exposed to excessive amounts of auditory stimulation. Again this can be regarded as a welfare issue.

It is important that all pets are exposed to a variety of situations when young, a commonly recognised fact when we consider the socialisation of dogs and cats (see *Chapter 6*). In the case of smaller pets, gentle handling when young can habituate them to being picked up and stroked. Owners need to be aware of how to handle their pet. For example, reaching into a cage and picking up a hamster (which may have been woken up by such an intrusion) can lead to defensive biting if not done with consideration. To a hamster, being picked up from above is similar to the swooping of a predator and is likely to initiate the anti-predator tactic of turning onto its back and biting. Such repeated treatment may well lead to increased aggression as the animal becomes more, rather than less, fearful. This is exacerbated by the pressure from the human hand, especially the enthusiastic grabbing of a child, which is likely to be quite painful if the ribs or abdomen are squeezed. A better approach would be to train the hamster to perceive handling as a positive experience. This can be easily achieved by placing small bits of food on the palm of the hand and allowing the

animal to climb on to the hand. Initially this should be done within the safety of its cage and later by gently holding it when it is on the hand and lifting it out of the cage. Likewise, the traditional means of picking a rabbit up by the ears, or a rat by its tail, is almost certain to produce an animal which is wary of being handled. Again, training the animal to approach and be picked up in such a manner that its body weight is continually supported by the handler will ensure less stress for both animal and human.

Some pets, rabbits for instance, do seem to perceive humans as threats to their territory. This is particularly noticeable during the breeding season when an otherwise docile animal can become aggressive. Many male rabbits are castrated or destroyed for this change in behaviour. Yet a consideration of the animal's ethology and biology can often rectify the problem. Provision of 'safe' areas, such as a piece of pipe for the animal to hide in and 'occupational therapy' in the form of activity foods, such as suspending apples and carrots from the roof of the cage, can help. Rabbits, like many mammals, spend much of their daily time eating. In the case of the rabbit, its digestive system has evolved to extract the maximum amount of nutrition from low-quality feed.[29] Many commercial diets provide high-quality feed in a concentrated form, thereby reducing the time the animal spends foraging and increasing its energy intake. These factors in combination can lead to increased activity and aggression. Reducing the feed quality, by providing hay

CIRCULATION FIGURES FOR POPULAR PET MAGAZINES		
Species	**Circulation to nearest 1,000**	**Example**
Dog	161,000	*Dogs Today; Our Dogs*
Cat	27,000	*Cats; Cat World*
Fish	91,000	*Practical Fishkeeping*
Birds + Rabbits	63,000	*Cage and Aviary Birds*
General	52,000	*Wild About Animals*
(Media: *Guardian* 17 January 1994)		

as forage, can substantially reduce these problems.

Unlike most dogs, cats and horses, many small pets spend their entire lives in the same environment, the confines of their cage. In contrast, the natural environment, terrestrial or aquatic, is one of constant and varied stimulation, albeit dominated by the need to be vigilant for predators. For all species, and especially the opportunistic rodents, the sterile conditions of cage life poses questions concerning the psychological welfare of these pets.[11] As discussed for horses, animals maintained in environments which are sub-optimal may develop stereotyped behaviours.[32] These behaviours can indicate an environment which is barren and restrictive in some way, for example a lack of tunnelling opportunities for caged rodents.[39] Alternatively, stereotypies may be indicative of some other unavoidable source of fear or stress[32] such as constant sound. Some owners try to provide their pets with stimulation such as an exercise wheel, which they perceive as positive and rewarding. Pet hamsters, rats, mice and gerbils can spend considerable portions of their daily activity cycle running in these wheels. It has been assumed that this is a positive activity and not indicative of a welfare problem. Yet it would seem that wheel running can be a stereotyped behaviour, often resulting from social or environmental deprivation.[39] Gerbils maintained in a semi-natural environment with the opportunity to burrow, forage, gnaw and nest build, as well as wheel run, showed significant differences in their behaviour compared to solitary animals kept in normal caged conditions.[39] For example, the isolated animals tended to be nocturnal rather than display the more diurnal activity pattern shown by the other group. There were also significant differences in wheel running. Solitary animals ran at speeds up to 2000 revolutions per hour, exceeding 20,000 revolutions per day, running for hours on end with only brief pauses. In dramatic contrast, the animals housed communally in a semi-natural environment rarely stayed in the wheel for more than a few revolutions at a time and never reached speeds above 50 revolutions per hour. These findings suggest that wheel running is a stereotyped activity indicating a sub-optimal environment.

In recent years there has been an increase in research being conducted on the behaviour and welfare of laboratory, farm and zoo animals[12,32,40] and how their lives can be enriched and their welfare improved. The findings of these studies will increase our knowledge of the social and physical requirements of these animals, many species of which are also kept as pets. The findings of such studies need to be made available to the pet-owning public in order to improve the lives of the many millions of animals we keep as pets and which enhance our own lives in so many ways.

References

1. Anthony, D. Telegin, T. Y. and Brown, D. (1991) The origin of horseback riding. *Scientific American*, **265,** 94–100.
2. Barclay, H. B. (1980) *The Role of the Horse in Man's Culture.* J. A. Allen, London.
3. Bergler, R. (1988) *Man and Dog: The Psychology of a Relationship.* Blackwell Scientific Publications, Oxford.
4. Bergler, R. (1989) *Man and Cat: The Benefits of Cat Ownership.* Blackwell Scientific Publications, Oxford.
5. British Horse Society (1992). *The Manual of Stable Management. Watering and Feeding.* Kenilworth Press, Buckingham.
6. Broom, D. M. and Kennedy, M. J. (1993) Stereotypies in horses: their relevance to welfare and causation. *Equine Veterinary Education*, **5,** 151–154
7. Brown, D. (1984) Personality and gender influences on human relationships with horses and dogs. In *The Pet Connection: Its Influence on Our Health and Quality of Life.* Eds. R. K. Anderson, B. Hart and L. A. Hart. pp. 216–223. Center to Study Human–Animal Relationships and Environments, University of Minnesota, Minneapolis, USA.
8. Caine, N. G. (1992) Humans as predators: observational studies and the risk of pseudohabituation. In *The Inevitable Bond.* Eds. H. Davis and D. Balfour. pp. 357–364. Cambridge University Press, Cambridge.
9. Clutton-Brock, J. (1992) *Horse Power: A History of the Horse and the Donkey in Human Societies.* Harvard University Press.

10. Cohen, E. (1994) Animals in medieval perceptions: The image of the ubiquitous other. In *Animals and Human Society: Changing Perspectives*. Eds. A. Manning and J. Serpell. pp. 59–80. Routledge, London.

11. Dawkins, M. S. (1988) Behavioural deprivation: A central problem in animal welfare. *Applied Animal Behaviour Science*, **20**, 209–225.

12. de Kock, L. L. and Rohn, I. (1971) Observations on the use of the exercise-wheel in relation to the social rank and hormonal conditions in the bank vole (*Clethrionomys glareolus*) and the Norway Lemming (*Lemmus lemmus*). *Zeitschrift fur Tierpsychologie*, **29**, 180–195

13. Engel, M. (1994) Just crackers about that chihuahua. *The Guardian*, January 17.

14. Frape, D. (1986) *Equine Nutrition and Feeding*. Longman Scientific and Technical, Essex

15. Fraser, A. F. (1992) *The Behaviour of the Horse*. C. A. B. International, Oxon, UK.

16. Fraser, A. F. and Broom, D. M. (1990) *Farm Animal Behaviour and Welfare*. Bailliere Tindall, London.

17. Hunt, S. J., Hart, L. A. and Gomulkiewicz, R. (1995) The role of small animals in social interactions between strangers. *Journal of Social Psychology*.

18. Jones, B. (1983) Just crazy about horses: The fact behind the fiction. In *New Perspectives on Our Lives with Companion Animals*. Eds. A. H. Katcher and A. M. Beck. pp. 87–111. University of Pennsylvania Press, Philadelphia.

19. Kavanau, J. L. (1967) Behaviour of captive white-footed mice. *Science*, **155**, 1623–1639

20. Kennedy, M. J., Schwabe, A. E. and Broom, D. M. (1993) Crib-biting and wind-sucking stereotypies in the horse. *Equine Veterinary Education*, **5**, 142–147

21. Kidd, A. H., Kelley, H. T. and Kidd, R. M. (1984) Personality characteristics of horse, turtle, snake and bird owners. In *The Pet Connection: Its Influence on Our Health and Quality of Life*. Eds. R. K. Anderson, B. L. Hart and L. A. Hart. pp. 200–206. Center to Study Human–Animal Relationships and Environments, University of Minnesota, Minneapolis, USA.

22. Klaus, M. H. and Kennell, J. H. (1976) *Maternal–Infant Bonding: the Impact of Early Separation or Loss on Family Development*. C. V. Mosby, St Louis.

23. Lawrence, E. A. (1984) *Rodeo: An Anthropologist Looks at the Wild and the Tame*. University of Chicago Press, Chicago, USA.

24. Lawrence, E. A. (1985) *Hoofbeats: Studies of Human–Horse Interactions*. Indiana University Press, Bloomington, USA.

25. Lawrence, E. A. (1988) Horses in society. In *Animals and People Sharing the World*. Ed. A. N. Rowan. pp. 95–115. University Press of New England, Hanover, USA.

26. Lawson, T. (1994) Stuck on sticks. *BBC Wildlife*, **12**, 40–44

27. Lewis, L. D. (1982) *Feeding and Care of the Horse*. Balliere Tindall, London.

28. McKay, J. (1991) *The New Hamster Handbook*. Blandford.

29. McBride, E. A. (1988) *Rabbits and Hares*. Whittet Books.

30. Macdonald, D. (1984) *The Encyclopaedia of Mammals*. pp. 482–485. George Allen and Unwin, London.

31. Mader, B., Hart, L. A. and Bergin, B. (1989) Social acknowledgements for children with disabilities: Effects of service dogs. *Child Development*, **60**, 1529–1534.

32. Mason, G. J. (1991) Stereotypies: a critical review. *Animal Behaviour*, **41**, 1015–1037

33. Messent, P. R. (1983) Social facilitation of contact with other people by pet dogs. In *New Perspectives on Our Lives with Companion Animals*. Eds. A. H. Katcher and A. M. Beck. pp. 37–46. University of Pennsylvania Press, Philadelphia.

34. Nowak, R. M. (1991) *Walker's Mammals of the World*. Vol. 2, 5th edn. The John Hopkins University Press, London.

35. Paul, E. S. and Serpell, J. A. (1993) Childhood pet-keeping and humane attitudes in young adulthood. *Animal Welfare*, **2**, 321–337

36. Platts, E. (1991) Out of the slime. *BBC Wildlife*, **9**, 420–423

37. Rees, L. (1984) *The Horse's Mind*. Stanley Paul, London.

38. Riddick, C. C. (1985) Health, aquariums and the non-institutionalised elderly. In *Pets and the Family*. Ed. M. Sussman. *Marriage and Family Review*, **8**, 163–173.

39. Roper, T. J. and Polioudakis, E. (1977) The behaviour of mongolian gerbils in a semi-natural environment, with special reference to ventral marking, dominance and sociability. *Behaviour*, **LXI**, 207–237

40. Stauffacher, M. (1992) Group housing and enrichment cages for breeding, fattening and laboratory rabbits. *Animal Welfare*, **1** (2), 105–127.

41. Tiegs, W. E. and Burger, I. H. (1993) Nutrition of horses. In *The Waltham Book of Companion Animal Nutrition*. Ed. I. Burger. pp. 97–109. Pergamon Press, Oxford.

42. Tyler, S. J. (1972) The behaviour and social organization of the New Forest ponies. *Animal Behaviour Monographs*, **5**(2), 85–196.

43. Veevers, J. E. (1985) The social meaning of pets: Alternative roles for companion animals. In *Pets and the Family*. Ed. M. Sussman. pp. 11–30.

44. Waring, G. H., Wierzbowski, S. and Hafez, E. S. E. (1975) The behaviour of horses. In *The Behaviour of Domestic Animals*. 3rd edn. Ed. E. S. E. Hafez. pp. 330–369. Bailliere Tindall, London.

CHAPTER 10

The End of a Relationship: Coping with Pet Loss

JUNE McNICHOLAS and GLYN M. COLLIS

Introduction

It is inevitable that for most pet owners there will come a time when they will have to cope with the loss of a pet. For some owners, the death of a pet may be a very stressful event; for others such a loss may have little significance in their lives. The aim of this chapter is to examine responses to the loss of a pet and what might be done to help, especially if responses are severe. We consider why reactions to pet loss can vary and explain why we feel that pet loss may not best be considered a form of bereavement. We discuss the nature of the stress that may be a consequence of pet loss and how this relates to the involvement of a pet in a person's lifestyle and the nature of the relationship between the owner and the pet, especially where the pet may have been a valuable source of support.

The loss of a pet may be viewed as a stressful life event with the degree of impact it causes dependent upon the degree of disruption caused to the owner's life. This, in turn, is dependent on the role and functions served by the person–pet relationship. In a small proportion of cases the severity of disruption can be equivalent to that caused by bereavement and appropriate forms of intervention may be necessary. However, for the general population of pet owners, the effects of loss are likely to be of a lesser impact and require a different kind of intervention, if any. We distinguish between **uncomplicated pet loss** and **complicated pet loss** and try to identify circumstances in which complicated pet loss may occur.

We also discuss some special aspects of pet loss that may contribute to anxiety, such as euthanasia, enforced pet loss and circumstances where the loss of a pet exacerbates existing problems. We examine the issue of helping children understand the loss of a pet. Although we are primarily focusing on the loss of a pet through death, it is recognised that many of the responses may occur through loss under other circumstances, such as theft or straying.

Understanding Pet Loss

There is considerable variation in the nature of person–pet relationships and the role pets play in the life of their owners. This should lead us to expect considerable variation in the range of responses to the loss of that relationship from the death of the pet. It is important that we accept and seek to understand the individuality of the person–pet relationship in order to cope with reactions to pet loss, whether within ourselves or in others.

Two extremes in person–pet relationships and responses to pet loss are clearly apparent. On the one hand large numbers of pets are abandoned and it is clear that for a proportion of pet owners parting from a pet is of little importance, causing no more disturbance to their life than the discarding of an unwanted object. There may even be pleasurable relief at the absence of the pet. On the other hand, many owners go to considerable lengths to retain their pets in difficult circumstances and there is growing evidence that, for some pet owners, the loss of a pet can cause very marked distress. Between these extremes there is an enormous variety in reactions to pet loss.

It is common for the loss of a pet to be regarded as a 'bereavement'. While this may be appropriate in some instances, it is not likely to represent the wider population of pet owners. One reason for this is the wide variation in the responses to pet loss. Also, in some cases, the more intense reactions to pet loss are not solely (or even mainly) caused by the loss of the pet — we refer to this as complicated pet loss.

Further reservations are that careless use of the term bereavement in this context is likely to be seen as insensitive and possibly offensive to those who have suffered the loss of a close family member or a similar human relationship. Moreover, there is a danger that health professionals might perceive the term as being used carelessly, with the consequence that the real problems of pet loss are taken less seriously than they should be. Finally, applying a label such as bereavement may lull us into thinking that we have a better understanding of pet loss than is really the case, with implications for how we attempt to alleviate the consequences of pet loss.

What is Lost when a Pet Dies?

Why is it that pet owners differ so much in their responses to pet loss? The answer lies in the nature of the relationship formed. Within this broad statement, we can isolate a number of overlapping components which, at one time or another, have been used to characterise close person–person relationships and which seem to have a particularly significant role in person–pet relationships:

- the emotional nature of the relationship;
- the support that some pets provide seems to help their owners cope with stress;
- the companionship provided by pets;
- the role a pet plays in everyday routines and lifestyle of the owner.

Typically literature has referred to the person–pet relationship in terms of 'attachment'. However, this term does not fully descibe the person–pet situation. In its narrow technical meaning, an attachment refers to the close relationship of a young child to a parent based on feelings of security.[6] In a penetrating discussion of the application of the concept of attachment to adult relationships, Ainsworth[1] suggests that a subset of adult human relationships are properly regarded as affectional bonds if they are based on a long-enduring affectional tie that is maintained during absences and where the partner is important as a unique individual. Typically, separation will cause distress and loss will cause grief. However, only a subset of affectional bonds are attachments; the criterial feature of an attachment is the experience of security and comfort in the presence of the partner. The distinction between attachment and affectional bonds is well illustrated by Ainsworth's insistence that a mother's bond to her child is not properly called an attachment because, typically, she does not gain security from the child, however much the child may gain security from her. It seems very unlikely that security is particularly important in most person–pet relationships. In making this claim we distinguish between: (i) security as it is experienced when a dog acts as a deterrent or defender against mugging or burglary and (ii) security in the sense of a non-specific feeling of being at ease and psychologically comfortable because of the proximity of a particular person, a feeling that is not tied to any specific threat. It is the latter sense that relates to the concept of attachment. Since it is unlikely that security is a dominant feature of most person–pet relationships, we conclude that, generally, it is not helpful to characterise person–pet relationships as attachments.[10]

Although the concept of bereavement is often associated with the concept of attachment, we would argue that it is more useful to view pet loss within the framework of psychosocial stress caused by the loss of a relationship and its roles and functions for the owner. The degree of disruption to the owner's emotional, social and physical functioning caused by the loss of a pet influences the response and explains the variation. Stress enters the picture in two ways. First, the loss itself causes stress, both emotionally and because of the changes to the owner's routines and lifestyle. Secondly, the person–pet relationship may have performed some functions which supported the owner against other potential sources of stress, support which is no longer available after the loss.

Functions and Roles in Relationships — Pets as Sources of Social Support

The concept of social support is well established in psychology as a mechanism to explain some of the variability in human responses to stressful events. It has been found that persons who have strong supportive relationships with others, which they can turn to at times of stress, may be buffered against minor stressors or better able to cope with major stressful events. Supportive relationships have been found to enhance recovery from physical illness such as stroke,[17] myocardial infarction[13,26] and cancer[50] and also to protect against some of the mental distress and physical reactions to adverse events such as a bereavement.[27] Since pet ownership has been found to be associated with recovery from, or decreased risks of, cardiovascular disease[3,14] and has also been found to alleviate stress arising from bereavement,[2,5] it is plausible that there are strongly supportive functions derived from the person–pet relationship.

Social support is a generic concept, which can be subdivided in a number of ways: it is commonplace to distinguish emotional support, esteem support, network support and instrumental support. Figure 10.1 illustrates the known functions and benefits of social support derived from human relationships.

Many of the descriptions of the benefits derived from pet ownership bear a strong resemblance to accepted definitions of the effects of perceived emotional social support e.g. the belief that one is cared for, loved, esteemed and valued.[9,21] It is argued that the effects of person–pet relationships and their benefits to physical and psychological health should be investigated within the framework of perceived social support and its known influence on positive health outcomes. The fact that pets are not human may be advantageous in that they are predictable and relatively unchanging in their affection and there is no fear that the relationship will be damaged by displays of weakness or emotion, or by excessive emotional demands.

Emotional support from pets may be inferred from the consistent evidence that pets are perceived to reduce loneliness and they may be sought out in times of stress and talked to by their owners. In the role of confidant, pets are non-judgmental and predictable in their positive feedback of their owners' worth and anything said will remain confidential. **Esteem support** may be afforded in the person–pet relationship through the position of power and control held by the owner. Unlike human relationships, which may be undermined by external stressors that threaten esteem such as unemployment, financial difficulties or loss of status, the person–pet relationship is rarely affected by such events, remaining constant, predictable and rewarding with the owner in control. **Instrumental support** from pets is rather less obvious but refers to the provision of tangible services such as when a dog is a house guard, or the control of vermin by cats. Service dogs, such as guide dogs, hearing dogs and assistance dogs for disabled people, also perform valuable instrumental functions in providing increased mobility and independence. Other functions of an

KNOWN FUNCTIONS AND BENEFITS OF SOCIAL SUPPORT FROM HUMAN RELATIONSHIPS				
Type of support	**Provisions**	**When sought**	**From whom**	**Known benefits**
Emotional support	Fulfilment of the need to feel cared for, loved and important to someone.	Specific close relationships turned to when stressful life events provoke fear or threat requiring demonstration of comfort and expression of love/regard by others.	Usually close affective relationships e.g. partner, closest friend, close relative in regular contact.	Alleviation of stress arising from major stressors such as bereavement[27]. Significant predictor of good prognosis in recovery from physical illness such as stroke[17] and cancer.[50] Availability of close confiding relationship particularly important to stress resistance.[19,20]
Esteem support	Reassurance of competence and worthy of respect from others. Fosters self-respect and self-worth. Provision of knowledge of being needed and valued by others.	When events threaten self-esteem, e.g. failure, unfavourable social comparison, sense of being useless to anyone.	Usually but not exclusively close relationships. Partner, family and friends important but may also turn to others who are able to demonstrate their need/respect for your role.	Low self-worth can heighten vulnerability to depression. Esteem support important in alleviating some stress arising from events threatening sense of self-worth such as unemployment,[48] or through altered body image such as mastectomy or physical disability.
Instrumental support	Availability of practical assistance with some task. Availability of advice or service.	When one needs tangible assistance or particular advice.	Does not have to be a close relationship, and may not include any emotional component. Can be casual requests for help, the recognition of help routinely given, or the seeking of specialist assistance in connection with major stressor.	Provides sense of others' involvement and willingness to help. Protects against stress of coping alone.
Network support	Sense of belonging to a social group. Regular contact with others reduces sense of isolation.	Not especially sought in response to the presence of a stressor. No particular purpose or goal to be met.	Does not have to be a close relationship and may not include any emotional component. Casual friendships, team members, co-workers who may also fulfil companionate roles.	Social isolation known to heighten vulnerability to depression and illness.
Companionship	Recreation, relaxation, naturalness, spontaneity, pleasurable shared activities.	Not especially sought in response to the presence of a stressor. For pleasurable ends only, with no particular purpose or goal to be met.	Does not have to be a close relationship and may not include any emotional component. Casual friendship, team members, co-workers.	Elevates general psychological well-being and may protect against minor stressors through fostering positive mental health.[41,42] Does not have a significant effect on alleviation of major life stressors.

FIG. 10.1: The known functions and benefits of social support derived from human relationships.

instrumental nature may be the use of pets as social statements, where a certain type of pet creates an image for its owner they perceive as desirable, or a symbol of success. **Network support** is a measure of one's regular contact with others. Social isolation, which is the lack of a social network, is known to exacerbate depression and contributes to a higher incidence of morbidity and mortality. Pets are known to be powerful social catalysts, facilitating interactions even between relative strangers.[29,33] Pet ownership may also broaden a social network by prompting membership of clubs and societies concerned with animals. **Companionship** is seen as theoretically distinct from social support.[40,41] It does not offer extrinsic support but provides intrinsic satisfactions such as shared pleasure in recreation, uncensored spontaneity, play and relaxation. Such activities are pursued for their own sake, rather than for a specific purpose such as solving a problem. They are seen as fulfilling a need for pleasurable involvement with others. Companionship may be important in fostering positive mental health, whilst social support may be important in preventing threats to mental health.

Of all the benefits attributed to pet ownership, companionship is perhaps the most widely accepted. Pets do afford pleasurable company, the opportunity to play in ways that adults are often unable to do, except with small children, for fear of embarrassment. It is perhaps the elements of companionship and enhanced network support that explain reported increased measures of psychological well-being and physical health.[43]

The Role of the Pet in the Owner's Lifestyle — Degree of Impact

The more integral the pet is in a person's daily life activities, the closer the relationship, or the more important the functions of the pet, then the greater the degree of social and emotional disruption that loss of the pet will cause and the greater the adjustment required to life without the relationship. The closeness of a relationship between two persons can be viewed in terms of the interdependence between two people as revealed in the frequency, intensity and diversity of their impacts on each other and the period of time over which these impacts continue.[23] This formulation can easily be extended to person–pet relationships. Most owners regard their pet as a family member, living in the same household and involved in family routines. This impact is usually strong, both in emotional investment and behaviour and may be frequently conducted in a range of diverse activities enacted together. Since the person–pet relationship is essentially predictable, the pattern of interconnected activities and interactions is even more likely to be characterised by stability than in many human relationships. In addition, as some pets may live with their owners for 10–15 years, the pattern is likely to be enduring over time.

Thus, a proportion of person–pet relationships may be legitimately regarded as close relationships. We stress **some** since it is likely that not all person–pet relationships are characterised by all the ingredients of a close relationship. Some may be purely recreational with little perceived support derived from the relationship. Even those that do contain elements of closeness are usually regarded as less significant than the human relationships in a person's life.

In summary, a successful person–pet relationship may be viewed as one where the perceived benefits of the relationship outweigh the costs and responsibilities of pet ownership. The benefits may be simple pleasure in owning the animal and in companionship, but there may be stronger elements of support from the relationship and a high degree of involvement of the pet in a number of routines important to lifestyle. The greater the pet's involvement in the relationship, the greater the stress that may arise from its loss. This stress may arise from: (i) the loss of a relationship in which one had a degree of emotional investment; (ii) the disruption to lifestyle routines; (iii) the awareness that a valued source of support has become unavailable with the loss of the pet; (iv) heightened vulnerability to the effects of actual external stressors. In general, the loss will be more stressful if it is perceived to be uncontrollable or unexpected.

The Experience of Pet Loss

Here we outline our reasons for suggesting that in the majority of cases the term 'bereavement' is not applicable to pet loss. In doing this we must first briefly examine some of the terms in common use in the bereavement literature. **Bereavement**, in its narrow theoretical sense, is the state which follows an actual or perceived loss of a valued object, state or relationship.[8] Although most usually applied to the loss of a human relationship through death, it has been extended to the loss of employment, loss of a home, loss of a limb through amputation and loss of health.[37,44,40,48] What constitutes a bereavement (and so sanctions the right to grieve or mourn), is culturally defined and carries with it the expectation that the experience will result in a considerable behavioural, psychological or physical impact on the bereaved person, which will often necessitate social and emotional adjustment.

Grieving is a reaction to bereavement, but a reaction that is part of the process of accepting and adjusting to the loss. Accounts of the grieving process emphasise progression through stages or transitions, each being different from the preceding or succeeding one, toward a resolution.[36] It is regarded as a functional process whereby the emotional energy spent in grieving is gradually withdrawn and invested in acceptance of the new circumstances and the formation of new relationships. **Sorrow** is also a reaction to bereavement and, emotionally, is similar to grief. However, it is not a process that is worked through with qualitative changes on the way to achieving a resolution. Rather, it is more accurately a single-symptom state[8] which, after an intense phase, will usually fade away. **Mourning** is the outward expression of the grief and sorrow that arise from a bereavement. The acceptable contexts and expected behaviours of mourning are culturally defined. Whilst there is considerable variation from culture to culture, the ritualisation of death is almost universal and prescribes conventions for the behaviour of the deceased's family and periods of mourning before it is acceptable to reinvest in another relationship.

Pet loss is not culturally recognised as a state of bereavement, nor is it clear that there is a case for doing so. Our reasons are, first, that it is not clear that the responses to pet loss generally or widely fit those responses associated with a bereavement. Some studies have demonstrated that the responses to pet loss can bear striking similarities to responses to bereavement, such as social withdrawal, disturbances to sleep and appetite, prolonged sadness and crying, disturbances to concentration, experiences of increased physical illness and belief that one sees or hears the lost one. However, studies that document such severe reactions to pet loss are mainly drawn from populations who have been referred to counselling services after the death of a pet,[38,49] have a history of other psychological difficulties,[22] or are undergoing other stressful life events, such as moving to a residential care home for the elderly.[31] Therefore, considerable caution should be exercised in extrapolating the findings of such research to general populations.

Studies that have looked at reactions to pet loss amongst a more representative sample of pet owners have failed to find such strong responses to loss. One study found similarities between pet loss and human bereavement in emotional reaction, but not in intensity or in duration.[4] There is also evidence that death of a pet does not predict depressive symptoms whilst death of a human does.[39] Pet loss is a very frequently occurring stressor in mid-life families (occurring twice as frequently as the next most frequent event — children leaving home), but the death of a family pet is perceived as less stressful than the death of an immediate family member or a close friend.[16] Gender differences in stress response found in other studies of family stress[35] are also apparent: 40% of wives reported that pet death was 'quite' or 'extremely' disturbing, compared to 28% of husbands.[16] There was no indication from that study that husbands were understating their responses, nor that 'disturbing' was the same as experiencing a bereavement.

Our second reason for not regarding pet loss within a bereavement model is that bereavement itself comes under a wider heading of stressful life events, which have varying levels of risk for stress responses and require varying levels of social and emotional readjustment. Not all of these stressful life events are losses and not all are severe. In general, stress is greatest when the degree of change brought about by an event is greatest. If a relationship, human or otherwise, is of particular importance (either because of the degree of involvement in a substantial number of aspects of daily life, or because of particular functions it served that are not perceived as available in other relationships), then the more the loss is felt and the more difficult it is to cope without that relationship. Loss of a close human relationship, such as a partner or close friend, is particularly associated with disruptions to lifestyle and to social, emotional and psychological functioning, with temporary consequences for psychological and physical health.

Pet loss, in a minority of cases, may cause severe disruption to lifestyle, but for the majority of pet owners, the loss may be emotionally disturbing but is not likely to be significantly disruptive. Death of a pet is unlikely to involve the degree of disruption that death of a close human relationship involves. Routines, for the most part, remain intact, financial and social circumstances are not usually subjected to significant alteration and existing social relationships remain largely unchanged. For these reasons we see pet loss as an event that may exert a degree of emotional, social or physical disruption commensurate with the roles and functions that the relationship afforded, but to which adjustment is less likely to be a problem than a bereavement. This is not to say that pet owners do not feel sorrow or distress at their loss, most will probably experience a variety of responses, but they will not be as lasting or intense as other major losses.

Pet Loss and Grieving

Similarly, in examining the process of grieving, we question whether grieving accurately describes the general reaction to pet loss. Intuitively we may assume that most pet owners grieve when a valued pet dies or is lost to them. However, this may not be true. If we consider grief as a process of psychosocial transitions that require resolution in order to attain readjustment, do pet owners generally have to negotiate those stages or processes, or are they experiencing the more unitary state of **sorrow** rather than **grief**? Again, it is probably dependent on the degree of disruption caused by the pet loss. If acceptance of the loss is particularly difficult, or if the loss requires major revision of social and behavioural routines and emotional investment (to the extent that lifestyle has to be restructured) it may well be appropriate to describe the responses to pet loss as a grieving process. If there are no substantial changes to these dimensions, no transitions that have to be made and no 'new' environment to which to adjust, then the responses could more accurately be described as sorrow. Although the feelings of sorrow may be intense, there is no negotiation of stages or processes of change. Over time the sorrow diminishes, though essentially unchanged in nature apart from the reduction in intensity, until it has passed. It may re-emerge at times of particular remembrance such as anniversaries or in familiar routines or places where the pet was involved, but the tenor of one's life is not unduly disturbed.

The distinction between sorrowing for a pet and grieving for a pet is of more than academic interest. If we are to understand the responses to pet loss, develop ways of helping owners adjust to loss, or persuade practitioners (both medical and veterinary) to recognise pet loss as a psychosocial stressor; we need to provide both a framework in which to place that understanding and recognition

THREE LEVELS OF PET LOSS			
Level of pet loss	Pre-loss state	Impact of loss	Responses	Interventions
Non-complicated loss	Moderate or satisfactory existing relationships, routines and socio-emotional functioning. Pet may be included in this but not in a central or major role.	Unlikely to cause significant disruption to existing routines, relationships, or socio-emotional functioning.	Similar to the unitary (non-phasic) state of sorrow. Crying, feelings of sadness, thoughts of death, wanting time alone or a day off work, etc. May be intense over a short time. Fades with occasional re-emergence on events provoking memories, e.g. anniversaries.	Professional intervention not essential. Owners may contact helplines or support groups for reassurance of normality and social acceptability of responses.
Loss complicated through stress overload	Concurrent or pre-existing stressors putting pressure on exising relationships, routines or socio-emotional functioning, e.g. divorce, unemployment, recent human loss, physical or mental illness.	Further disruption to relationships, routines and socio-emotional functioning. Increased pressure on already strained coping strategies.	Increased risks for stress reactions, e.g. elevated vulnerability to depression, anxiety, which may be manifested as physical symptoms leading to higher incidence of physical illness.	Intervention required to reinstate strategies for coping with pre-existing problems and with pet loss, e.g. stress management counselling, medical or psychological referral.
Loss complicated by high emotional dependency on pet and/or centrality of pet in lifestyle	Existing relationships, routines or socio-emotional functioning highly dependent on pet involvement. Close human relationships may be fragile or absent.	Severe disruption to many aspects of normal functioning requiring major readjustment to absence of pet.	May be similar to the state of bereavement. Responses may follow phases of transitions associated with grieving. Severe emotional responses, cognitive disturbance, social withdrawal, depression, elevated risk of morbidity.	Intervention required to help psycho-social transition to readjustment to life without the pet e.g. professionally qualified grief counselling, psychiatric or psychological referral.

FIG. 10.2: Three levels of pet loss.

and the identification of appropriate coping mechanisms required to deal with it. If the loss of a pet causes emotional distress but has little impact on normal social and emotional functioning, with most predominant lifestyle routines remaining intact, it may be best viewed as uncomplicated pet loss. This may well require reassurance that such reactions as crying, preoccupation with the death for a short time, feelings of blame and sadness, are normal, but it would be inappropriate to couch such reassurances in terms of bereavement counselling.

However, whilst the term bereavement is probably not generally applicable to pet loss, practitioners should recognise that some instances of pet loss can result in substantial disruption to social and emotional functioning. This may be almost indistinguishable from bereavement of a more accepted nature and will produce responses needing stages or psychosocial transitions to be negotiated in order to attain adjustment. A response of this nature should be viewed as complicated pet loss and may occur for a variety of reasons, some of which are discussed below. Complicated pet loss will need intervention of a more specialised nature than uncomplicated pet loss. This may require not only some form of grief therapy but also investigation of possible underlying problems that have exacerbated or contributed to the response. In Fig. 10.2 we identify three models of pet loss where roles and functions of the relationship and integration of the pet into lifestyle, may differentiate complications to pet loss.

Pet Loss and Mourning

If most other major losses are marked by culturally defined and accepted rituals of mourning, this cannot be said of pet loss, whether complicated or uncomplicated. This is of particular concern. Even where pet loss is not seriously disruptive to normal life, owners frequently express the need to talk about their experience and to have their feelings recognised and accepted by others.

Sadly, outward expressions of grief and sorrow are not generally condoned by society. There are no accepted rituals for the passing of a pet, no recognised period of mourning and no accepted time when a new pet may be acquired. In fact, many owners are particularly distressed at the reactions from others to their experience of pet loss. Even close friends or relations may be unwilling or unable to understand the depth of feeling that an owner feels when a special pet is gone. Others may assume that a quick replacement of a pet, as one would replace a household article, is the solution, neglecting to recognise the emotional components of the distress. Pet owners wishing to engage in some sort of ritualisation of death, such as the use of pet crematoria or a printed obituary, often face ridicule or total lack of understanding, even by their closest human companions. Many, therefore, feel embarrassed and unable to reveal what they feel.

This lack of permission to express grief or sorrow openly has been referred to as '**disenfranchised grief**',[12] which can place an added burden on the loss experience itself. Doka[12] cites pet loss as one instance of disenfranchised grief for which society effectively denies permission to express feelings openly. He sees a need for recognition that pet loss can produce distress and a need for people to express their feelings freely.

Special Aspects of Pet Loss

Euthanasia

Although not necessarily a predictor of severe responses to loss, the responsibility for deciding when to end life can be problematic and anxiety-provoking. In general, most owners are happy to accept veterinarians' opinion that levels of constant pain, presence of disease with little chance of satisfactory recovery, or greatly diminished quality of life for the pet through old age or chronic illness merit euthanasia. Literally translated, euthanasia means 'easy death' and most pet owners consider the last kindness they can show their pet, even their obligation under the relationship, is to provide painless release from suffering. For some, this can even be a comfort in the loss, knowing that they did the 'right thing' and ensured their pet was spared a death that could be prolonged or traumatic for both owner and pet.

For others, euthanasia can result in guilt for having passed a death sentence. They may experience constant doubts that it was unavoidable, belatedly wish for a second opinion, or blame a veterinarian for making a diagnosis that their pet could not recover. There may also be a problem when the need to euthanase is completely unexpected by the pet owner, having not realised the seriousness of their pet's condition.

Most veterinarians are aware of the conflict facing pet owners whose pets are to be euthanased, the wish to keep the pet and the responsibility to do the right thing. Indeed, we should not assume that veterinarians themselves are free from all of the effects of pet death. They too can feel distressed at the death of an animal they have been treating, perhaps since its youth. In general terms, most veterinarians recognise that it is important to discuss why it may be kinder to euthanase the pet rather than to continue treatment, when and where to carry it out and whether the owner should be present during the procedure. Wherever possible, the owner should be involved in these decisions. Some less acute cases may be safely deferred for a day or two so that family members all have their own chance in their own way to bid farewell to the pet. Some owners may prefer to have their pets euthanased at their home, especially if the animal has shown distress at visiting the veterinarian's surgery. A special meal or a last cuddle and an easy death in the pet's own familiar surroundings should be an option and may greatly ease the pet owner's distress.

One area where veterinarians and owners may experience disagreement is whether the owner should be present during the procedure or should wait elsewhere until called to view the body. Some owners are unable to face the thought of watching their pets die, others

wish to be present to ensure that the pet dies easily and to be reassured that it is dead. Similarly, some veterinarians prefer the owners to be absent, being aware that some animals gasp, twitch or empty both bladder and bowels as they expire, and this can have an effect on the owner. Other veterinarians encourage the owner's presence, seeing it as less distressing for the pet than being handled by strangers. Again, the choice must be individual. If the owner has the procedures adequately explained and knows what to expect, there should be no reason why they should not be present if they wish. Even if the owner is not present they should have the opportunity to see the body after euthanasia has been carried out. This ensures that they see the animal at peace and reassures them that the procedure was carried out promptly.

The rituals surrounding death vary between cultures but, in western cultures, owners may be asked if they wish to take the pet's body home for private burial in a favourite spot in the garden, or whether they wish the veterinarian to arrange cremation and return of the ashes to the owner. Some veterinarians have access to areas used as pet cemeteries where headstones or memorials can be erected. These can be very comforting to the owner, both as a lasting reminder and as recognition of their feelings.

Tactfully handled, euthanasia can become a comfort to the pet owner. Less gentle dealing with the situation can result in lasting distress.

Enforced Pet Loss

Sometimes the choice of ending a relationship is imposed by external forces. The prohibition of pets by housing associations and in some residential homes is a frequent cause of an involuntary end to person–pet relationships. Unfortunately, the pet owners who are most likely to be caught up in this problem belong to vulnerable groups, for example older people. In our society, ageing can diminish both the quality and quantity of social and emotional transactions, producing a shrinkage of the social network so that emotional investment in the person–pet relationship can be high. The move to any residential care establishment is likely to be stressful in itself, requiring major adjustment to lifestyle. The loss of a valued relationship that may have been an emotional focus in its own right, a reminder of absent or deceased family members, or a prominent feature in daily routines, can be a considerable added stressor. This loss may result in more negative feelings to the move, difficulties in adjusting to new routines and diminished sense of physical and psychological well-being.[31]

The main source of the problem of enforced pet loss is one of recognition. There is a widespread assumption that residential homes will not accept personal pets or will be unwilling to help find alternative arrangements for the pet, with the result that many pets are euthanased unnecessarily. Moreover, older people themselves may be unwilling to disclose their worries about losing a pet for fear of appearing foolish. Most importantly, residential care establishments often fail to recognise the importance of pets to some people. In a recent survey[11] only 20% of homes for older people and 5% of homes for children or people with learning difficulties reported having any written policy on pets. Where policies did exist there was no reference to procedures for investigating pet ownership prior to entry, to the referral of potential residents to homes that allowed pets, or to ways of assisting in making mutually satisfactory arrangements for the pet. Owners of cats and dogs were especially vulnerable to enforced pet loss with fewer than a quarter of all homes being prepared even to consider permitting them.[30]

The problem is widespread; animal welfare shelters in six cities reported to a survey that up to 1500 pets, again the majority being cats and dogs, were placed with them each year because owners were going into residential care.[11] There is a further unknown number of pets euthanased by vets and many unclaimed animals from temporary 'welfare boarding' cases whose owners are discharged from hospital into residential care homes. In many cases there is additional distress for the owner since they are not consulted about the future of their pet. The solution is to promote wider recognition of the problem and inclusion of the issue in formal written policies of those responsible for managing residential care facilities.[32]

Children and Pet Loss

The greatest proportion of pet owners are in families where there are children and the death of a family pet may be the first experience of death a child may encounter. The pet may or may not have been a major part of the child's life, but the struggle to understand the concept of death may be problematic. A commonly cited reason for owning pets is to help educate children in responsibilities towards others and on issues of birth, sex and death, but experience shows that many parents shield children from the death of a pet. Parents may go to great lengths to withhold information from a child that a pet is very ill and should be euthanased. Untrue explanations for the pet's absence may be given, such as 'going to live in the country'. This may afford no comfort since children are distressed if their pets are given away.[7] Euphemisms such as 'being put to sleep' may alarm the child, who may wonder 'If I go to sleep will I not wake up?' We would argue that the child should receive explanations that are accurate and commensurate with their ability to understand the nature of death.

There is considerable uncertainty about the nature and development of young children's understanding of death, but it is fairly clear that by the age of 5–7 years the majority of children understand that (i) death is an irreversible state; (ii) death involves the cessation of all life functions; and (iii) death is inevitable for all living things.[45]

Up to the age of about 5 years, children construct reality through their own limited experience. Death is not always seen as irreversible[24] or may be confused with states of sleep, going away, or a type of illness.[34] Cause and effect relationships are not established at this age and children may invoke some pre-logical or egocentric explanation for events. The death may be believed to have been caused by some unrelated behaviour by themselves or others. For example, if they have been naughty on the day that the pet died, or it was the day someone visited, they may see one as the cause of the other. Self-blame and guilt can occur when a child attaches this sort of explanation to a death and may lead to disturbed behaviour when the death is recalled.[15] It would be cautionary to explain that the pet death was not the fault of anyone and to be patient if the child repeatedly questions about the pet in their efforts to understand.

In older children there may be school or learning problems, or preoccupation with the deceased.[25] Occasionally there may be more overt depressive symptoms or manifestation in physical illness such as stomach aches, headaches, etc. In the vast majority of cases these will be short-lived, but parents should be aware that such symptoms could be attributable to the loss of a pet and the struggle to understand the event. In adolescents there is also the possibility that reaction to pet death could be associated with syndromes such as lack of energy, eating disorders or even substance abuse.[18]

Children should be involved in the situation when a family pet dies. Explanations should be as clear as possible and repeated if required. Euthanasia should be discussed beforehand; the opportunity to say a last farewell may be much appreciated and the shock less severe than coming home from school to find the pet inexplicably but permanently absent. Children of all ages may appreciate some concrete recognition of the loss; a bunch of flowers or a 'funeral' can all help, as can exercises of compiling a list of the nice things about their pet and their favourite memories of the pet.[47]

Reactions to Pet Loss as a Symptom of Other Losses or Problems

Pet loss may cause particular distress if other stressors are present in the owner's life. Relationship difficulties, other losses, or unresolved problems in the owner's life may exacerbate the effects that pet death may produce. This may operate in two ways. First, the existing problems may have shaped the relationship with the pet into one where the pet assumes emotional centrality for the owner, perhaps to the relative exclusion of other meaningful or trusted relationships. In this context the response to pet loss is likely to be severe and will at least in part be due to whatever earlier difficulties have remained unresolved. Keddie[22] documents several cases where difficulties with human relationships caused emotional dependence upon a pet. Death of the pet then resulted in what he has described as **pathological mourning**, this being prolonged intense grief which required psychiatric intervention to resolve the earlier problems and those caused by the death of the pet. Similarly, Stewart[46] reports the phenomenon of **double bereavement** where a pet was jointly owned with a deceased partner. The presence of the pet as a way of retaining established routines and as a source of invested memories of the partner when alive, can help the surviving partner to cope with the human death. However, when the pet dies, the loss is not only of the pet but of the routines previously shared with the deceased partner and of the focus of memories associated with that time. Responses to the pet death are then likely to incorporate many losses that were not dealt with at the time of the earlier death. Again, intervention may be required to aid recovery from the accumulated losses centred on the loss of the pet.

A second way in which pet loss may be particularly severe is the simultaneous influence of other stressors in the owner's life. Stress can be seen as cumulative and the presence of many stressors may diminish coping strategies that may otherwise be adequate for one or two stressors. Loss of a relationship, a home, financial difficulties, work or health problems, may be already imposing considerable strain on an owner. Death of a valued pet may not be easy to bear in the face of other negative influences in life and is unlikely to be dealt with in isolation from all the other problems.

It is also important to note that pet loss may be masking a more serious problem. It is well known for clients of doctors, counsellors, psychologists and psychiatrists to present with one particular problem, often the most easily articulated, only to disclose later the real reason for their seeking help. Pet loss counselling services, where offered, should be aware that some people presenting with problems of pet loss have a hidden agenda and hidden needs. Pet loss may be the easiest problem for them to express, or pet loss counsellors be perceived as the least threatening of available sources of advice, but it may not be the help they require. Great care should be taken in identifying these people and seeking their referral to medical, psychological or psychiatric services.

Alleviating Pet Loss

There may well be considerable emotional distress even among those people for whom the loss of a pet does not seriously disrupt their daily life. A pet's position in an owner's life may not be fully appreciated until it has gone and it is common for the pet owners themselves to be bewildered by the intensity of their feelings, sometimes to the extent that they doubt their responses to be normal. They may also be angry or shocked at the absence of any understanding from those around them. In short, they may experience the disenfranchisement of expression that Doka[12] describes. For these reasons there is the need for some guidance for alleviating distress, whether severe and complicated or relatively uncomplicated.

For most owners experiencing distress, just the knowledge and recognition of what is 'normal' or commonplace will be of considerable help in reassuring them that their experience is not isolated, abnormal or even psychotic. Literature describing common reactions to pet loss is to be welcomed. There is a pressing need for a variety of easily available, easily readable books and pamphlets that can reassure owners that it is quite normal to experience reactions such as crying, feelings of sadness, mood swings and temporary disruptions to sleep and appetite. Many people also experience frequent unbidden thoughts of the pet, dreams, difficulties in concentration, or the need to take time off work because they feel so unhappy. It is common to feel that one might have been in some way to blame for the pet's death, or could have done more. These are symptoms of psychosocial stress that can occur when pressures or stressful life events hit us. They are common, accepted and recognised as responses to sudden and/or relatively major stresses, whatever these may be. There is no need for guilt or fear to be felt when an owner unexpectedly finds that they are experiencing any of these responses. Unless they persist to the point where normal life is disrupted or existing relationships become threatened by the responses or conflict arising from them, there is little for the pet owner to be alarmed about.

Some such guides do exist and are invaluable to those owners who want to work through their distress alone. It is not every one who wishes to talk openly about their feelings. Veterinarians, psychologists and other professionals should seek to ensure that information about coping with pet loss is available to those that need it.

Ritualisation

Some pet owners wish for some ceremony or recognition of their pet's death. This does not necessarily indicate the presence of severe responses or profound difficulties in accepting the death. At a simple level it may merely indicate the wish to recognise the pet's life in some preferred way other than the anonymous impersonal alternatives of disposal. In addition to the cremation services offered by an increasing number of veterinary practices, there are specialised pet crematoria. These crematoria will deal sensitively with the disposal of the body, with options for individual cremation and headstones if requested, as well as collective cremation with the ashes being put in a garden of remembrance. Some crematoria offer counselling or just an opportunity to talk about a pet. Pet owners should not be deterred by the views of others from using these services if that is what they feel would help them. It is a decision they have a right to make and few seem to regret. Some owners see it as a lasting memorial; others view the ceremony attached as a final celebration of the pet's life.

Pet owners may also wish to record their pet's life in an obituary. The authors have noted that a number of specialist journals for pet owners offer this service. The readership will be mostly sympathetic and of like mind and publication will be seen as granting permission to express the feelings of loss. Other owners may wish for a memorial that is less like a human ceremony. Pledges of donations to favoured charities, or a plaque on a pen in an animal rescue centre can fulfil this role and provide a sense of comfort in a valued service being performed as an act of remembrance.

A Change in Thinking

Whilst it is usual for pet owners to concentrate on the loss, much can be gained if they can gradually turn their thoughts to the pleasures they gained from owning the pet. This is a method adopted by counsellors, but it can be successful on a self-help basis too. Concentration on the pleasing memories, the humorous episodes, games or holidays with growing children and the way the pet fitted into the family, can be comforting. Such thoughts may help the relationship to be viewed as a total experience, so that overall, ownership of the pet was a positive experience. Few people would wish they had never owned their pet because of the feelings they had when it died.

Many pet owners want, even need, to talk of their pet, its death and their reactions to it. So far we have discussed the ways in which an owner may wish to deal with the loss on their own. Literature, remembrance rituals and positive thinking can all play their part, but some owners may need contact with others, perhaps outside the family, either because all the family is similarly affected by the death or because they want external reassurance that what they experience is normal.

Help From Veterinary Staff

Veterinarians and veterinary nurses can provide a valuable first contact for owners, especially if their pet was being treated recently. The veterinary profession is becoming increasingly aware of the need to be sympathetic and to make time to discuss the owner's feelings. Veterinary nurses and technicians, too, are being trained in the recognition of the effects of pet loss. Owners should be encouraged to feel that their veterinarian's surgery is approachable for discussions about their reactions to the loss. Although veterinarians and veterinary nurses will only be able to provide sympathy and clarify factual matters surrounding the pet's death, this may be all that is required in instances of uncomplicated pet loss to meet the owner's needs. However, if an owner is displaying intense emotional distress, or the veterinary staff have reason to believe that further help is required, it is recommended that they advise the owner to seek professional advice through their family doctor. Such owners may feel happier going to their family doctor if they are doing so on the advice of another professional or because it gives them an opening line: 'my vet said I should come to see you'.

Pet Loss Helplines

Mader and Hart[28] describe the process of setting up such a telephone helpline in the USA, modelled on a successful telephone helpline for people contemplating suicide. Manned by volunteers from a veterinary school, the line received over 500 calls in its first year. Most were callers distressed after losing a pet which they had owned for a long time, 12 years or longer for cats or dogs. Not all pets were dead; some callers appeared to experience distress over their elderly pet's declining health and wanted to speak of their concerns over their possible reaction when it died. Euthanasia was mentioned in the majority of calls; 45% of callers had had their animals euthanased and 17% were considering it. Guilt about pet death was also a frequent reason for calling. Most callers made only one call, which suggests that they felt a need for a listening ear and reassurance, rather than a need for counselling or active support. Most believed themselves to be receiving adequate or strong support from friends or relatives, suggesting that they were not without people they could turn to; use of a helpline seemed to be an added aid in their distress.

At the time of writing, the Society for Companion Animal Studies has recently set up a similar helpline in the UK to be manned by volunteer 'befrienders'. There may also be a role for self-help groups; many callers to the American helpline requested, or were referred to, such groups but these are not common in other countries. Such groups could provide a forum for owners to discuss their feelings, reassure themselves that they are not alone and to help each other find ways of coping with their distress. However, if most owners experiencing uncomplicated pet loss only require reassurance that theirs is not an uncommon experience, the turnover of people attending such groups might be too high for the group to be viable so that a helpline is a more realistic alternative.

Although there is much to be commended in helplines and support groups, there are caveats that should be noted. Most users are likely to be experiencing relatively uncomplicated reactions requiring sympathy and reassurance, but some may not be so uncomplicated. As mentioned earlier, it is possible for the responses to pet loss to cause or mask more serious problems. Instances of complicated pet loss are likely to require intervention beyond that available through helplines, and, in our view, training should be given to identify those people who should be strongly recommended to consult their family doctor.

Symptoms that should alert volunteers to the need for professional help for these

people include: intense psychological and physical symptoms arising from the time of loss, low perceived availability of social support from friends and family, a considerable degree of disruption to social and emotional functioning, a history of mental illness, recent or concurrent additional stressors such as divorce, death of a close human relationship, employment difficulties and medical illness.

Family Doctors

Many owners may think of approaching their family doctor, but may be uncertain of whether they will be treated sympathetically. Advice from veterinarians to consult a doctor can help considerably, being seen as the advice of one professional that it is acceptable to approach another. In any case, if an owner feels that they are not getting over the loss as quickly as expected, or are experiencing physical symptoms such as sleeping or eating problems, or just feeling unwell, a family doctor should be consulted. Family doctors are not as dismissive as one might think, although there is still a need to ensure that the medical profession is supplied with information to help acceptance of pet loss as a stressor. Doctors are also becoming increasingly aware of the effects of stress on health and, with the knowledge of an owner's medical history, they should be able to advise on appropriate helping strategies. Family doctors are also able to refer people to a trained counsellor — many have counsellors attached to their practice — or to the local psychological or psychiatric services, as appropriate.

Help From the Voluntary Sector

Owners who are already experiencing stressful circumstances such as relationship problems, unemployment or a bereavement in the family and who are already in contact with one of the many appropriate support organisations (such as those offering relationship guidance, or bereavement counselling, or one of many support groups for medical conditions), should not be afraid to discuss with their counsellor any added difficulties arising from the pet loss. Owners who have not yet contacted such an organisation may feel that now is the time to do so and receive help for the pre-existing stressor and the more recent pet loss which may have exacerbated their distress. There may also be counsellors, who will be able to help, in the workplace or through organisations for the well-being of particular groups such as elderly people. However, it is envisaged that the standard course of action is to consult the family doctor.

Replacing a Pet

There can be no guidelines on the best time to acquire another pet; it is an individual or family decision. Although many owners feel unable to invest in another relationship quickly after a pet has died, others may find replacing a pet a welcome distraction. Both are valid viewpoints. It seems that most people eventually do acquire another pet unless there are particular reasons why they cannot. Pet ownership is frequently an aspect of a chosen lifestyle and so a new pet is almost inevitable. For those embarking on the new relationship, the time can be a mixture of pleasure and painful memories: pleasure at the growth of the new relationship, painful memories of the previous pet. The new pet is a new partner in a relationship, as unique as the previous one, and they should not be compared.

References

1. Ainsworth, M. D. S. (1989) Attachments beyond infancy. *American Psychologist*, **44**, 709–716.
2. Akiyama, H., Holtzman, J. M. and Britz, W. E. (1986) Pet ownership and health status during bereavement. *Omega; Journal of Death and Dying*, **17**, 187–193.
3. Anderson, W. P., Reid, C. M. and Jennings, G. L. (1992) Pet ownership and risk factors for cardiovascular disease. *Medical Journal of Australia*, **157**, 298–301.
4. Archer, J. and Winchester, G. (1993) Bereavement following death of a pet. *British Journal of Psychology*, **85**, 259–271.
5. Bolin, S. (1987) The effects of companion animals during conjugal bereavement. *Anthrozoös*, **1**, 26–35.
6. Bowlby, J. (1969, 1973, 1980) *Attachment and Loss. Vol. 1. Attachment. Vol. 2, Separation, Anxiety and Anger. Vol. 3, Loss, Sadness and Depression.* Penguin Books, Harmondsworth.
7. Bryant, B. K. (1990) The richness of the child–pet relationship: a consideration of both benefits and costs of pets to children. *Anthrozoös*, **3**, 253–261.
8. Clegg, F. (1988) Bereavement. In *The Handbook of Life Stress, Cognition and Health.*, Eds. S. Fisher, and J. Reason. pp. 61– 74. Wiley, New York.
9. Cobb, S. (1976) Social support as a moderator of life stress. *Psychosomatic Medicine*, **38**, 300–314.
10. Collis, G. M., McNicholas, J. and Morley, I. E. M. (1993) Can pet–person "attachment" explain the beneficial effects of owning pets? In *Proceedings of the International Congress on Applied Ethology, Berlin 1993*. Eds. M. Nichelmann, H. K. Wierenga, and S. Braun. pp. 365–367. Humboldt University, Berlin.
11. Collis, G. M., Morley, I. E. and McNicholas, J. (1993) Pets and people in residential care. *Social Care Research Findings No.44.* Joseph Rowntree Foundation, York.
12. Doka, K. J. (1989) *Disenfranchised Grief: Recognising Hidden Sorrow.* Lexington Books, Lexington.
13. Fontana, A. F., Kerns, R. D., Rosenberg, R. L. and Colonese, K. L. (1989) Support, stress and recovery from coronary heart disease: a longitudinal causal model. *Health Psychology*, **8**, 175–193.
14. Friedmann, E., Katcher, A. H., Lynch, J. J. and Thomas, S. A. (1980) Animal companions and one year survival of patients after discharge from a coronary care unit. *Public Health Reports*, **95**, 307–312.
15. Furman, E. (1974) *A Child's Parent Dies.* Yale University Press, New Haven.
16. Gage, M. G. and Holcomb, R. (1991) Couple's perception of stressfulness of death of the family pet. *Family Relations*, **40**, 103–105.
17. Glass, T.A., Matchar, D. B., Belyea M. and Feussner J. R. (1993) Impact of social support on outcome in first stroke. *Stroke*, **24**, 64–70.
18. Gudas, L. J. (1993) Concepts of death and loss in childhood and adolescence. In *Children and Disasters*. Ed. C. F. Saylor. pp. 67–84, Plenum Press, New York.
19. Hobfall, S. E. and Lieberman, Y. (1987) Personality

and social resources in immediate and continued stress resistance among women. *Journal of Personality and Social Psychology*, **52**, 18–26.

20. Hobfall, S. E. and Walfisch, S. (1984) Coping with a threat to life: a longitudinal study of self-concept, social support and psychological stress. *American Journal of Community Psychology*, **16**, 317–331.

21. House, J. S. (1981) *Work Stress and Social Support*. Addison-Wesley, Reading, MA.

22. Keddie, K. M. G. (1977) Pathological mourning after the death of a domestic pet. *British Journal of Psychiatry*, **131**, 21–35.

23. Kelley, H. H., Berscheid, E., Christensen, A., Harvey, J. H., Huston, T. L., Levinger, G., McClintock, E., Peplau, L. A. and Peterson, D. R. (1983) *Close Relationships*. Freeman, New York.

24. Koocher, G. P. (1973) Childhood, death and cognitive development. *Developmental Psychology*, **9**, 369–375.

25. Koocher, G. P. (1986) Coping with a death from cancer. *Journal of Consulting and Clinical Psychology*, **54**, 623–631.

26. Kulik, J. A. and Mahler, H. I. M. (1993) Emotional support as a moderator of adjustment and compliance after coronary artery bypass surgery: a longitudinal study. *Journal of Behavioral Medicine*, **16**, 45–63.

27. Littlewood, J. (1992) *Aspects of Grief: Bereavement in Adult Life*. Routledge, London.

28. Mader, B. and Hart, L. A. (1992) Establishing a model pet loss support hotline. *Journal of the Americal Veterinary Medical Association*, **200**, 270–274.

29. McNicholas, J., Collis, G. M., Morley, I. E. and Lane, D. R. (1993) Social communication through a companion animal: the dog as a social catalyst. In *Proceedings of the International Congress on Applied Ethology, Berlin 1993*. Eds. M. Nichelmann, H. K. Wierenga and S. Braun. pp. 368–370. Humboldt University, Berlin.

30. McNicholas, J., Collis, G. M. and Morley, I. E. (1993) *Pets and people in residential care: towards a model of good practice*. Final report to the Joseph Rowntree Foundation, October 1993.

31. McNicholas, J., Collis, G. M. and Morley, I. E. (1993) *Psychological and physical effects of enforced pet loss*. Paper presented to Conference on Pets, Health and Quality of Life for Older People, Edinburgh, September 1993.

32. McNicholas, J., Collis, G. M. and Morley, I. E. (1994) *Guidelines: People in Residential Care — The Need for Policy on Pets*. Joseph Rowntree Foundation, York.

33. Messent, P. R. (1983) Social facilitation of contact with other people by pet dogs. In *New Perspectives in our Lives with Companion Animals*. Eds. A. H. Katcher and A. M. Beck. pp. 37–47. University of Pennsylvania Press, Philadelphia.

34. Nagy, M. (1948) The child's theories concerning death. *Journal of Genetic Psychology*, **7**, 3–27.

35. Olsen, D. H. and McCubbin, H. I. (1983) *Families: What Makes Them Work?* Sage Publications, Beverly Hills.

36. Parkes, C. M. (1971) Psychosocial transitions: a field for study. *Social Science and Medicine*, **5**, 101–115.

37. Parkes, C. M. (1972) The components of reaction to loss of a limb, spouse or home. *Journal of Psychosomatic Research*, **16**, 343–349.

38. Quackenbush, J. E. (1983) Pet bereavement in older owners. In *The Pet Connection: Proceedings of the Minnesota–California Conference on the Human–Animal Bond, 1983*. Eds. R. K. Anderson, B. L. Hart and L. A. Hart. pp. 292–299. University of Minnesota, Minneapolis.

39. Rajaram, S. S., Garrity, T. F., Stallones, L. and Marx, M. B. (1993) Bereavement — loss of a pet and loss of a human. *Anthrozoös*, **6**, 8–16.

40. Raphael, B. (1984) *The Anatomy of Bereavement: a Handbook for the Caring Professions*. Hutchinson, London .

41. Rook, K. S. (1987) Social support versus companionship: effects on life stress, loneliness and evaluations by others. *Journal of Personality and Social Psychology*, **52**, 1132–1147.

42. Rook, K. S. (1992) Social relationships as a source of companionship: implications for older adults' psychological well being. In *Social Support: An Interactional View*. Eds. B. R. Sarason, I. Sarason and G. R. Pierce. pp. 219–250. Wiley, New York.

43. Serpell, J. A. (1991) Beneficial effects of pet ownership on some aspects of human health and behaviour. *Journal of the Royal Society of Medicine*, **84**, 717–720.

44. Shukla, G. D., Cahu, S. C., Tripathi, R. P. and Gupta, D. K. (1982) A psychiatric study of amputees. *British Journal of Psychiatry*, **141**, 50–53.

45. Speece, M. W. and Brent, S. B. (1984) Children's understanding of death: a review of three components of a death concept. *Child Development*, **55**, 1671–1686.

46. Stewart, M. (1983) Loss of a pet loss of a person: a comparative study of bereavement. In *New Perspectives on Our Lives With Companion Animals*. Eds. A. H. Katcher and A. M. Beck. pp. 390–406. University of Philadelphia Press, Philadelphia.

Index